COMMUNICATION and HEALTH:
Systems and Applications

COMMUNICATION
TEXTBOOK SERIES
Jennings Bryant—Editor

Applied Communication
Teresa Thompson—Advisor

NUSSBAUM ● Life-Span Communication:
Normative Processes

RAY/DONOHEW ● Communication and Health:
Systems and Applications

COMMUNICATION and HEALTH:
Systems and Applications

Edited by

Eileen Berlin Ray
Cleveland State University

Lewis Donohew
University of Kentucky

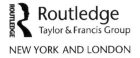

Routledge
Taylor & Francis Group

NEW YORK AND LONDON

First Published by
Lawrence Erlbaum Associates, Inc., Publishers
365 Broadway
Hillsdale, New Jersey 07642

Transferred to Digital Printing 2009 by Routledge
270 Madison Ave, New York NY 10016
2 Park Square, Milton Park, Abingdon, Oxon, OX14 4RN

Library of Congress Cataloging-in-Publication Data

Communication and health : Systems and applications / edited by Eileen
Berlin Ray, Lewis Donohew.
   p. cm. — (Communication textbook series. Applied
communication)
  Includes index.
  ISBN 0–8058–0154–5
  ISBN 0–8058–0697–0
  1. Communication in medicine. I. Ray, Eileen Berlin.
ii. Donohew, Lewis. III. Series.
R118.C615 1990
610′.141—dc19

89–30978
CIP

Publisher's Note
The publisher has gone to great lengths to ensure the quality of this
reprint but points out that some imperfections in the original may be
apparent.

This book is dedicated to:

George, Bryan, and *Lesley* and
to the memory of *Claire Devine Jordan*—EBR

And to the memory of *Ford* and
Ethel Couchman Donohew—LD

Contents

Contributors

JANE D. BROWN   Center for Research in Journalism and Mass Communication, The University of North Carolina at Chapel Hill, Chapel Hill, NC 27599

REBECCA J. WELCH CLINE   Department of Speech, University of Florida, Gainesville, FL 32611

LEWIS DONOHEW   Department of Communication, University of Kentucky, Lexington, KY 40506

EDNA F. EINSIEDEL   Communications Studies Programme, University of Calgary, 2500 University Drive N.W., Calgary, Alberta, Canada T2N 1N4

JOHN R. FINNEGAN, JR.   School of Public Health, Stadium Gate 27, 611 Beacon St., SE, University of Minnesota, Minneapolis, MN 55455

VICKI S. FREIMUTH   Department of Communication Arts and Theatre, University of Maryland, Baltimore, MD 21201

GARY L. KREPS   Department of Communication Studies, Northern Illinois University, DeKalb, IL 60115

KATHERINE I. MILLER   Department of Communication, Michigan State University, E. Lansing, MI 48824

KIMBERLY A. NEUENDORF   Department of Communication, Cleveland State University, Cleveland, OH 44115

EILEEN BERLIN RAY   Department of Communication, Cleveland State University, Cleveland, OH 44115

BRENT D. RUBEN   Office of the PhD Program, School of Communication, Information and Library Studies, Rutgers University, 4 Huntington St., New Brunswick, NJ 08903

TERESA L. THOMPSON   Department of Communication, University of Dayton, Dayton, OH 45469

K. VISWANATH   School of Public Health, Stadium Gate 27, 611 Beacon St., SE, University of Minnesota, Minneapolis, MN 55455

I

FOUNDATIONS

1

Introduction:

Systems Perspectives on Health Communication

Lewis Donohew
University of Kentucky

Eileen Berlin Ray
Cleveland State University

In 1975, the Health Communication Division of the International Communication Association was formed. Eleven years later, the Commission on Health Communication was formed by the Speech Communication Association. As health communication has become an area of specialty for communication scholars, more advanced courses are being offered at colleges and universities. Although a number of excellent introductory texts are available for use in lower division courses, there is a need for advanced and graduate-level texts in health communication.

The goal of this book is to meet that need. Specifically, it was designed to address theoretical and applied issues for understanding the health communication process across a number of contexts. It employs a systems framework to present relevant issues in the communication of health care ranging from micro to macro levels. This range includes an examination of factors affecting an individual's processing of information about health, and changes in uses of communication and its outcomes. These include interpersonal, small group, and organizational health-care contexts and factors involved in informing individuals about health through the mass media and other sources, both through public health campaigns and in the day-to-day climate of awareness and knowledge of health issues.

In the following pages, we define health communication, discuss relevant systems concepts, and offer a brief preview of their application in the forthcoming chapters.

DEFINITION AND RELEVANT SYSTEMS CONCEPTS

Health communication is the dissemination and interpretation of health-related messages. The disseminator may be an individual, an organization, or a mass medium. The interpreter may be an individual, a group, an organization, or an undiscriminated mass public.

A *system* is a set of components surrounded by a boundary that regulates the flow of inputs and a transformation into outputs. Within a health-communication context, these *components* are the individuals disseminating or interpreting the messages. The boundaries are arbitrary, resulting in the subsystems that provide the organizational framework and substance of this book. At the interpersonal level, they are tightly drawn to include relevant dyadic relationships in the health-care process, such as doctor–patient communication. As we expand the boundaries to include others directly involved in the provision of health care, we can examine the role of small groups in health communication, such as the health-care team. Further expansion of the boundaries enables us to consider the dynamics within the organizational context. Here we look at the interdependence between the health-care providers and the recipients of that care, as influenced by external structural considerations. Even further expansion of the boundaries brings us to mass communication systems in which an organization or organizations devoted to public surveillance—the mass media—collect and disseminate health information to a broad general public.

In all of the instances, the definitions of the systems involved are somewhat more complex and involve several *subsystems* that we describe in more detail later in this section. A general systems framework is advantageous for examining the dissemination and interpretation process in a number of ways. The concepts of particular relevance include input, throughput, output, interdependence, dynamic homeostasis, negative entropy, the principle of nonsummativity, equifinality, and feedback within both broad general systems and more specific cybernetic systems.

For our purposes, *input* refers to any messages or other sources of information coming into the system from its external environment. These messages are then translated and transformed by the components of the system—ordinarily, people—into a form that is useful for the system, which we refer to as *throughout*. The end product, after it has passed through the system, is called *output*. It is during this input–throughput–output process that the interdependence among the components of the system is especially critical.

By *interdependence,* we are referring to the fact that a change in any one component of the system will result in some degree of change in the remainder of the system. In the beginning, a system is confronted with some stimulus or situation requiring a response. This stimulus or situation may, in fact, be threatening to the system or it may offer some kind of positive opportunity. The system may respond by rejecting the stimulus, by adapting in order to accommodate it, or possibly by accommodating to part of it but leaving part of it unresolved. This unresolved portion may continue to be a threat or an unaccepted opportunity, so much so that it threatens the balance of the system and its ability to adapt to future stimuli. This is the process of *dynamic homeostasis,* the ability of a system to adapt while maintaining a state of balance.

As originally conceptualized, the *law of entropy* refers to the fact that all systems eventually run down. *Negative entropy* is information that helps the system impede that process and preserve itself. Here, when we refer to negative entropy, we are talking about the collection of information by a system that permits it to avoid chaos and disruption and to preserve itself. For example, a public health campaign about AIDS is intended to help a system, through acquisition of greater knowledge, to preserve itself in the presence of a major threat.

One of the most attractive features of the systems conceptualization is the *principle of nonsummativity,* which refers to the fact that the whole is greater than the sum of its parts. This means that the responses of the system to its environment are not limited to simple mechanistic actions based on the inputs from its various components, but are complex responses based on the *interaction* of those components. This is particularly relevant in conceptualizing health communication within a systems perspective. As the system boundaries expand and we move from the interpersonal to the group, the organization, and the mass levels, we have much more than the additive accumulation of each additional subsystem. What we have in each case is a new and unique set of dynamics that must be understood within their appropriate system contexts.

Equifinality refers to the fact that a goal may be reached by multiple paths and with multiple starting points. For example, an individual has just been diagnosed as having a treatable form of cancer. Her doctor recommends she see a specialist for treatment. Her family members also give her advice and seek information from their own sources. In addition, she gathers information from all available media sources regarding her particular cancer. For example, both the American Cancer Society and the National Cancer Institute are trying to decrease the incidence of mortality from breast cancer. Their goal is to catch breast cancer as early as possible. Some of the multiple path points include interpersonal channels for teaching women how to do self-examinations and urging some frequency of mammograms, and mass channels for disseminating printed material with information on self-examination and/or mammograms, and public service announcements. Multiple starting points vary, in part, depending on assumptions made about the audience. If it is assumed that the audience recognizes the importance of early detection, the interpersonal and/or mass channels will focus on behaviors that will increase the probability of early detection. However, if it is assumed that the audience is not convinced of the importance of early detection, the focus may be on informing them of warning signals and persuading them of the importance of early detection prior to discussing specific behaviors.

All of the systems concepts discussed previously fit under the umbrella of general systems theory. However, of critical importance is the ability of the system to regulate itself through the use of *feedback* it obtains from the external environment. This feedback loop serves a *cybernetic* function, resulting in *deviation counteracting* (negative feedback) or *deviation amplifying* (positive feedback) changes within the system. Counteracting feedback enables the system to maintain its steady state on the way to achieving its goals, while amplifying feedback enables the system to change, adapt, and grow. If adaptation or change puts the system out of balance, counteracting feedback can bring it back within acceptable parameters.

AN OVERVIEW OF THE CHAPTERS

As previously mentioned, this book is organized within an overall general systems framework. Subsystems are nested within larger systems, beginning with the interpersonal level and ending with the mass level. Part I of the book includes two chapters that provide a foundation for the rest of the volume. In this chapter, the editors lay out the relevant systems concepts emphasized throughout the remaining chapters. In chapter 2, Finnegan and Viswanath further elaborate on the systems framework in their discussion of medical and public health influences on the research agenda embracing both the interpersonal (medical) and mass (public health) areas of health communication.

Part II focuses on health communication within medical contexts. Dyadic systems are discussed in chapters 3 (Thompson) and 4 (Ruben). Both examine the interdependencies and cybernetic functions of the dyadic interaction in health-care settings. Thompson provides a thorough review of literature on provider–patient communication, and Ruben discusses issues of pathology, etiology, and treatment within this interpersonal context. The systems level is then expanded to the small group level in chapter 5 by Cline. Here we see how the expansion of system boundaries to the health-care team, as well as to informal and formal support groups, affect the dynamics of the health-care system. Boundaries are further expanded to the organizational level in chapter 6. Here Ray and Miller examine communication between members of the health-care organizations and the recipients of this care, as well as communication among the organization workers themselves. The complex dynamics of this communication is clear, as the dyadic and group levels are subsumed at this higher system level.

Part III further expands the system boundaries to the mass level. These chapters address efforts to reach audiences through the mass media and public education. Although we tend to think of these areas as operating at social systems level, it is not possible to classify public health campaigns at a single systems level. A closer look reveals a need for greater complexity. When we speak of mass media directed at a society, as do the chapters by Neuendorf; Donohew; Brown and Einsiedel; and Freimuth, or of health education, as does Kreps, we are describing a social systems level. However, when we speak of strategies for targeting and designing messages, as in social marketing or in the design of messages aimed at high- or low-sensation seekers, for example, we are talking about small group and even intrapersonal systems. Here it is the *individual,* rather than the mass public, that is the unit of analysis.

In chapter 7, Neuendorf provides an extensive review of health images in the mass media and describes the constellation of influences on individuals in the area of health, including the mass media, health organizations, health professionals, and other individuals.

Donohew, in chapter 8, concentrates on research leading to the design of targeted health messages—with emphasis on the effects of the biology of communication on attention to messages—and offers a model of information processing containing both cognitive and affective elements tested in general and in health communication settings.

In chapter 9, Brown and Einseidel describe a relatively recent development in public health campaigns—social marketing—which takes audience differences into much greater account in the design of the campaign. They provide a stage-by-stage description of the design and execution of contemporary campaigns, including the evaluation component.

In chapter 10, Freimuth discusses issues involving information gaps in which public information campaigns often widen the gap between the educated and more affluent and the poor and uneducated. She discusses how to target—and how not to target—the poor and disadvantaged and outlines concerns with social systems constraints that interfere with reaching major segments of society. She also discusses the quality of "ends" information on television, to which the uneducated are largely exposed, as opposed to "means" information—information about how to achieve desired ends, which is presented in print media, to which the educated are exposed.

Finally, chapter 11 by Kreps returns us to the joint consideration of the interpersonal and mass levels. Here, he integrates all of the systems levels and emphasizes their interdependencies in his discussion of the critical role of communication in health education.

This book substantially differs from other books embracing health and communication in that it focuses on health care from a communication perspective. Although other disciplines have examined some communication issues, their typical view can be likened to viewing communication as just one more variable among many. We advocate communication as *the* critical variable, essential for effective health care, and around which the other variables must revolve.

2

Health and Communication:
Medical and Public Health Influences on the Research Agenda

John R. Finnegan Jr.
K. Viswanath
University of Minnesota

The study of human communication processes and effects has combined with the study of almost every human endeavor, and health has been no different (Berger & Chaffee, 1987; Costello, 1977). The marriage of health and communication in a self-conscious interdisciplinary relationship is generally regarded to have occurred in the mid-1970s, although it was certainly a common-law relationship long before (Cassata, 1978; Costello, 1977). Like all scholarly intermarriages, the relationship between the two areas of study has been growing and changing albeit sometimes tenuously ever since the field became "official." Each has been involved in their separate "dominant paradigm" issues that have been affecting theoretical, research, and methodological aspects of their joint intellectual domicile. These issues include critiques of current level-of-analysis distinctions in communication effects and processes, as well as broadening conceptualizations of "health" as individual and collective behavior formed in community social and cultural settings.

These issues have practical ramifications for the field. As we see here, they lay the groundwork for more integrated analyses of the role of communication in health, as well as expand definitions of *health outcomes* and the traditional institutional settings within which such research has been conducted.

This chapter examines the relationship of communication and health in light of these developments, and—if the metaphor may be pressed

one more time—suggests that there are developing perspectives pushing the marriage in promising directions of mutual discovery.

FIELD DEFINITIONS

To date the field of health communication has been defined with greater
emphasis on communication than health per se. This is not surprising
because it was communication scholars who sought to exercise their
expertise in health situations rather than health experts who sought
to illuminate communication effects. Scholarly overviews have defined
the field mainly emphasizing processes and taxonomies reflecting the
issues, branches, and methodological perspectives of the larger field of
communication science.

For example, Costello (1977) noted that health communication is the
study of the process by which individuals acquire and convert event
data about health into meaningful or consumable information, the ends
of which are "those of adaptation." Cassata (1980) defined the field as
"the study of communication parameters (levels, functions, and methodologies) applied in health situations/contexts" (p. 584). Noting a lack of
generalizable theory, he offered a matrix separating communication
levels, functions, health contexts, and communication methodologies
indicating the many combinations of research parameters used to delin-
eate the field.

In a related approach, Kreps and Thornton (1984) defined health
communication as concerned with "human interaction in the health
care process" (p. 2), focusing on the needs of patients/consumers in
health-care settings, but also noting the levels at which communication
processes and effects may be examined (intrapersonal, interpersonal,
group, organizational, public and mass communication). In a later
work, Kreps (1988) stressed the field's focus on information about
health ("pervasive, ubiquitous, and equivocal") and how it is sought,
processed, and shared at different levels of human interaction. In an
effort to better connect communication with health outcomes, Reardon
(1988) emphasized the role of the field in studying how and under what
conditions communication may persuade and motivate people to adopt
healthier lifestyles and behaviors as a matter of health promotion and
disease prevention.

Pettegrew (1988) discussed the importance of context in communication about health, noting the "theoretical pluralism" of the field and
that health communication dynamics are not embodied sufficiently or
convincingly in only "information versus persuasion" perspectives. All
communication is contextually bound in situation and culture that

to a large extent pre-determine health outcomes. Unconvinced of the "inextricable" link between health and communication offered by information or persuasion perspectives, Pettegrew recommended a change in the field's conceptualization of "audience" to facilitate building such a link. That is, humans are above all culture-bound storytellers, which provides a frame of reference to impart and assimilate meaning. How, and under what situational conditions different "narrative" frames of reference are related to health outcomes may, in his view, better test and give legitimacy to health communication as a field.

It is the issue of legitimacy that has concerned many scholars working in the field. The concern takes several directions: specifying field boundaries and definitions; developing a body of theory and research that secures an "inextricable link" between the fields; and "curricularizing" a standard body of knowledge in advanced degree programs (Cassata, 1978; Costello, 1977; Pettegrew, 1988).

Such concerns are not unique to the study of health communication, of course, but in a slightly altered form concern the development of human communication studies as a "mature science." There are two basic critiques about the development of the larger field that bear on health communication. One, expressed recently by Berger and Chaffee (1987), holds that the study of human communication overall lacks a general theory to explain and predict "a wide range of communication phenomena." As a result, they observed, the study of human communication has been expanding but fragmenting along the lines of different levels of analysis (intrapersonal, interpersonal, organizational, intercultural, mass) as if each of these branches were conceptually distinct. They noted, too, that the field's fragmentation is furthered by rivalries within the academy that lay claim to different branches of human communication studies.

However, one person's theoretical fragmentation, it seems, is another's theoretical pluralism. A second critique of the larger field, voiced by Halloran (1981), holds that the research agenda has been constricted to some extent because of institutional influences that have excessively determined the kinds of research questions, perspectives, and the kinds of studies conducted. This has been the case particularly in mass communication studies, Halloran averred, in which the needs of Western mass media have heavily influenced research directions and contexts. Although not disfavoring scientific approaches that better integrate levels of analyses in communication effects and processes, Halloran proposed both increased critical and cross-cultural research to redress the balance.

Although these critiques are not inherently contradictory, they provide the context for a closer analysis of research in trends in health communication. As a hybrid field, it also certainly has expanded but fragmented into level-of-analysis based branches. Whether it may be expected to provide general theory that is lacking overall, is to beg the question of whether it is equal to the task any more than, say, political communication. But like its hybrid cousin, the development of health communication as a mature science not only depends on "communication," but on the definitional distinctions, boundaries, and rivalries concerning its counterpart: health. It is this first partner in the field that brings to bear a significant set of institutional influences on research directions that are not often acknowledged or explored sufficiently in discussing the field. These concern specifically the influences of the medical and public health sectors and competing approaches to the idea of "health." Some evidence about trends in health communication research helps to make these influences clearer.

RESEARCH THEMES

Although overviews of the field generally acknowledge the importance of a wide variety of situations and contexts in the study of health and communication, a review of recent trends in reported research reveals an emphasis on "health" as outcomes that occur in the professional medical sector, the product of the interaction of patients and health professionals (health-care team) in privatized relationships. To those working in the field, this comes as less than stunning news. But it is important to note nonetheless because the focus on health in the medical sector has heavily influenced the kinds of research questions asked and investigations conducted. Moreover, there are significant changes underway that are beginning to influence a whole new set of questions and investigations.

The authors searched four major databases for the years 1983 through 1987 seeking research citations under the rubric "health and communication," and several variants. The databases included MEDLINE (National Library of Medicine), one of the largest and most frequently used databases, including citations from some 3,200 journals worldwide; the Educational Resources Information Center (ERIC), a national network including 16 clearinghouses devoted to citations of relevance to educators; PsycINFO (PSYC), the major citation index of the American Psychological Association; and Sociological Abstracts (SOCA).

Such a search requires a few caveats. Databases reflect what people put into them. Decisions to classify research citations under certain headings are made both by database gatekeepers and by authors who provide keywords as guides. Not all citations with some bearing on communication and health necessarily will appear under the search rubric unless authors or gatekeepers so classify them. Research articles may be framed in such a way that they will be classified under other topic headings even though they may contain important communication aspects. In part, this reflects both the conventional use of keyword classifications and the extent to which authors identify themselves as working in a specific field. And, although we believe these databases are the most likely repositories for health communication citations, there are other, smaller, databases that may include citations not listed therein. In brief, our review of health communication research is a nonempirical review of themes and trends.

With these caveats in mind, we extracted 322 entries under the search rubric in the specified years, and grouped them according to their primary themes based on bibliographic keywords. Twenty-nine thematic categories emerged (Tables 2.1 and 2.2). We then separated them according to their primary institutional context: medical or public health sectors. Fifteen of the themes (Table 2.1), including 69% of the cited literature, focused on health communication in the context of the formal medical/health-care delivery system. Fourteen themes, including 31% of the citations, dealt with health communication outside the formal medical sector in some aspect of public health. By far the majority of citations in both institutional contexts were contributed by the MEDLINE database (about 73%), followed by PSYC (about 12%), ERIC (about 11%), and SOCA (about 4%).

Figure 2.1 compares annual trends of the five most frequently appearing themes. Studies of interpersonal interaction between health-care professionals and patients/clients in the formal health-care delivery system comprise the largest number of citations consistently across each year. The other four categories show less consistency year to year in the number of citations, but three of the four also are related directly to communication in the formal health-care delivery system. For example, the term *information systems* refers to the development and impact of computer and other medical information systems to improve service delivery. *Interprofessional relations* focuses on the interaction of health-care professionals for more efficient and effective system operation, and *professional training* involves research suggesting programs or approaches to teaching health-care professionals communication skills. Only one of the five leading categories—*health campaigns*—focuses on the study of health and communication in a context other than the formal medical/health-care delivery system.

This review supports previous thematic analyses in a number of aspects important to the study of health and communication. Research

TABLE 2.1
Health Communication Research Citations
in Four Selected Databases, 1983–1987
Medical Sector Context

	MEDLINE	*ERIC*	*PSYC*	*SOCA*
Health professional/ patient relations	58	—	3	4
Patient compliance	4	—	—	—
Quality of care	5	—	—	—
Health-care cost analysis	1	—	—	—
Health information systems	23	1	—	—
Marketing of health-care	11	2	—	—
Health-care policy analysis	1	1	1	—
Health professional relations	23	2	3	—
Health problems of professional groups	2	—	—	—
Use of health services	10	—	—	—
Clinical strategies and problems	15	—	—	—
Diffusion of technology/ health-care	8	1	—	—
Diffusion of health-care research findings	3	1	1	—
Education of health professionals	23	4	—	—
Other	3	2	—	—
SUBTOTAL	190	14	8	4

has been conducted largely in the context of the formal medical/health-care delivery system emphasizing interpersonal communication (between health-care professional and patient/client, or professional to professional) and with an applied emphasis of how changes or improvement in these dynamics may result in better communication to facilitate individual health outcomes. *Health campaigns* is the single major exception to these themes, which focuses on communication processes and effects outside the formal medical/health-care delivery system, often at the community or societal level.

Extracting from these trends, one may conclude that if the field of health communication has a dominant paradigm, it may be described thus: Communication about health occurs primarily in the formal health-care delivery system, between individual patients/clients who

TABLE 2.2
Health Communication Research Citations
in Four Selected Databases, 1983—1987
Public Health Context

	MEDLINE	ERIC	PSYC	SOCA
Risk communication	7	—	—	—
Health/life campaigns	20	5	17	3
Health campaign ethics	—	—	1	—
Community programs	5	—	—	—
Outreach programs	6	—	—	—
Science reporting	2	—	—	—
Public policy analysis	1	—	—	—
Health and communication theory and methodology	2	—	—	—
Health information sources research	1	2	2	2
Analysis of media content/ health	—	4	4	2
Mass media effects and health	—	3	5	2
Development of communication technologies	—	6	—	—
Information seeking/health	—	—	1	—
Other	3	—	—	—
SUBTOTAL	47	20	30	9

seek explanations and/or solutions to perceived symptoms and/or health conditions and individual health professionals trained to offer diagnosis, treatment, or other solutions to these symptoms/conditions. The effectiveness of the relationship and thereby the efficiency of the system may be enhanced to the extent that barriers to communication are mitigated, helping patients/clients to adopt recommended behaviors to alleviate the symptoms/conditions.

This dominant paradigm presumes both a formal institutional setting (the medical/health-care delivery system) and a set of largely interpersonal communication variables and processes driven by empirical sociopsychological or behaviorist perspectives.

PRIVATE AND PUBLIC MODELS OF HEALTH

There are, of course, historical reasons for this evolution (painted here necessarily in broad strokes). As social historian Paul Starr (1982) has pointed out, the United States early in this century adopted an individualized, personal model of health out of the interplay of forces

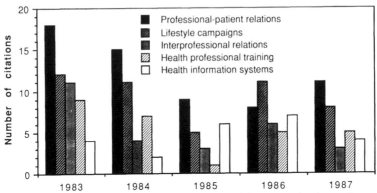

FIG. 2.1. Five most frequently appearing health communication topics in four databases from 1983 to 1987.

leading to the professionalization of medicine and to its dominance socially, politically, and economically of health and health care. Characteristics of this historical process included the organization of physicians into a potent political force to control who could enter the profession and generally how they should behave (licensing and disciplinary peer review), and the standardization of knowledge (medical school curricula). Moreover, governmental sanction for these functions in the form of quasi-public boards permitted the profession a visible "official" platform from which to exclude competing views of "health" (homeopathy, for example), as well as to control potentially competing models of health-care delivery (public health, for example). Starr noted that early in this century, the medical profession was successful in halting the expansion of a public health model of service delivery whose hallmarks were widespread availability of low-cost treatment, especially in major urban areas, and education for the prevention of disease. Public health efforts fell under the dominance of the medical profession, which succeeded in limiting their activities largely to treatment of the poor and indigent, and the control of infectious diseases that required some large-scale public action without which regular medical facilities might be overwhelmed.

In Starr's view, the development of public health as a field has been largely a debate about its mandate that was effectively limited early in this century because of the competitive threat it posed to the medical sector. As a result, public health has remained underdeveloped in the United States compared to other societies until only recently in this century.

The dominant paradigm of health arising from the privatization of health concerns focused on disease as a culturally defined anomalous or deviant condition that had behavioral ramifications for both patient and health-care provider (Parsons, 1951). Patients who perceived themselves as unhealthy were likely to exhibit "illness" or "sick-role" behavior (Bloom, 1963; Costello, 1977). The duty of the physician in the social context of the relationship was to reduce symptoms through diagnosis and treatment and to encourage patients to perceive themselves as recovering or rehabilitating.

Important changes began to occur after World War II that stimulated both medicine and public health to focus explicitly on the behavioral aspects of health. Epidemiology, the basic science of public health, began to amass a large body of quantitative evidence that strongly linked high levels of many adult chronic diseases to culturally induced behaviors. This was especially the case with heart disease, in which studies increasingly strengthened its connection to cigarette smoking; consumption of high-fat, high-sodium foods; untreated hypertension; obesity; and sedentary living (Keys, 1980). This emerging evidence pointed to the need for systematic approaches to primary prevention. In the context of privatized patient–provider relationships in the medical sector, the fields of preventive and behavioral medicine developed, drawing on the perspectives of psychology and social psychology. Research began to focus on the behavioral and psychological variables important to the process of prevention and adopting healthier behaviors, as well as on family and social environments as friendly or hostile to these goals (Somers & Weisfeld, 1986).

This same epidemiological evidence also suggested a set of strategies reaching far outside privatized patient–provider relationships. Mass levels of disease suggested the need for mass strategies of prevention. Moreover, because unhealthy behavior patterns were largely formed by social and cultural influences, some larger approach to intervention was required than could be provided in traditional privatized patient–provider relationships alone. The task was not only one of influencing individuals to change their personal risky habits, but of influencing change in the larger social and cultural environment that formed risky behaviors in the first place.

During the last two decades, these issues also have led to a rebirth of public health (sometimes called the second public health revolution; Green, 1986). They have both stimulated discussion of public health's mandate and expanded its scientific and applied purview in understanding and intervening in the causes and preventions of disease (Robbins, 1985; Terris, 1986). Unacceptable costs of medical treatment technology also have helped to more strongly cement the relationship between public health and preventive medicine. In part, this has resulted in the development of approaches to health that take the concept beyond disease-centered models per se.

EPIDEMIOLOGY AND HEALTH BEHAVIOR

Epidemiology—the science of public health—has developed an increasingly interdisciplinary focus on human behavior and its cultural and social influences as causes and prevention of disease. Research increasingly has aimed at the development of strategies making use of multiple levels of communication for mass intervention in behaviorally based disease processes. Cardiovascular disease was the first major target of this research because in most industrialized countries it is not only the leading cause of death, but is among the first to be linked strongly to socially and culturally influenced behavioral variables. Initial intervention research in Finland during the 1970s has been followed by major demonstration projects in the United States (California, Minnesota, Rhode Island, Pennsylvania), and worldwide (Blackburn, 1983; Elder, Hovell, Lasater, Wells, & Carleton, 1985; Farquhar et al., 1985; Mittelmark et al., 1986). These have been strongly influenced by a variety of fields including social marketing, community analysis and organization, and "empowerment" strategies as frameworks for the mobilization of communities and the management of social and behavioral change through lifestyle campaigns (Finnegan, Bracht, & Viswanath, in press). More is said about this later because it has particular bearing on integrating developments in the associated fields of health education and preventive medicine.

HEALTH BEHAVIOR AND COMMUNITY INTERVENTION

Although health education has been the primary professional link that bridges public health and preventive medicine, these developments have given rise to a new term with a somewhat larger purview: *health promotion*. Green (1986) described health promotion as "any combination of health education and related organizational, economic, and environmental supports for behavior conducive to health" (p. 1090). Health promotion is the "broader enterprise" including interventions affecting antecedent social and cultural conditions that spawn individuals' risky behavior, whereas health education focuses on the "voluntary participation of individuals in determining their own health practices" (Green, 1984, p. 186).

In this connection, Green (1984) noted the evolution of health education as a professional field from early pedagogic models of "information transfer" to a focus on behavior and associated contingent conditions. Models have developed to explain and predict individuals' health behavior and decision making in treatment, prevention, and rehabilitative contexts, taking into account both social and individual difference variables. In an extensive review of this literature, Becker and Maiman (1983) noted the extensive cross-fertilization of perspectives with varying emphases on social and individual difference variables. For example, Suchman (1966, 1967), influenced by a sociological perspective of the impact of social networks, suggested that there are strong links between membership and identification with certain social relationships and group structures that influence decisions to seek medical treatment and engage in preventive behaviors. Focusing on decision making about health under conditions of uncertainty, the Health Belief Model has emphasized perceptions and motivations as the primary predictors of health behavior (Janz & Becker, 1984). Langlie (1977) combined elements of both perspectives to explain and predict preventive health behavior as a function of perception variables (vulnerability, benefits, salience, self-efficacy), membership in different types of social networks (marriage, family, kinship, neighborhood, religion) and socioeconomic status. In an anthropological approach to how individuals process information about health, Fabrega (1977) emphasized the interrelationship of individuals' biological influences, social relations, phenomenological and memory processes. Others, such as Green (1986), have suggested that health behavior may be examined from the diffusion of innovations perspective that emphasizes characteristics of adopters, innovations, and source and situational conditions. This perspective in particular takes a somewhat more macroscopic perspective on the social and environmental conditions encouraging or mitigating the adoption of healthier behaviors as well as variables of individual difference. Moreover, as Chaffee (1975) explained, differing rates of diffusion may be examined as a function of external and internal communication "pressure" causing diffusion to accelerate or decelerate in relation to the normative S-shaped pattern of diffusion.

In practical terms, the intervention research outlined earlier provides fertile ground for integrating health-behavior research perspectives with the role of communication at multiple levels of interaction. What is frequently misunderstood about such research is that, as currently configured in the United States, it does not use merely "mass media" campaigns in seeking to influence unhealthy lifestyle patterns. Such research is not defined primarily by the channels it uses, but by the overall social framework within which people live, work, and interact: the community. What has been emerging in this research, under the influence of preventive medicine, behavioral epidemiology, and the applied approach of health education, is an integrated approach to prevention that is community centered. The rationale underlying the integration of these approaches to prevention is that social and cultural influences are crucial in learning and adopting behavior patterns and that they are importantly experienced by individuals through social aggregates and networks that make up communities (Eisenstadt & Shachar, 1986).

Three themes unify these views about the process of seeking social and behavioral change in health. First is the emphasis on powerful social and cultural forces influencing individuals' behavior (Blum, 1981). Communities form individuals' behavior symbolically and tangibly (Allen & Allen, 1987). As agents of the dominant culture, communities transmit values and norms that symbolically circumscribe some behavioral choices and encourage others. As systems of exchange and influence relationships, communities establish opportunities for people to behave in some ways, but not in others.

Following from this, a second common theme holds that communities themselves may be mobilized to act as change agents in the process of achieving social and behavioral outcomes in health. Mobilizing communities to act as change agents means that they both give local legitimacy to values and norms for healthy behaviors and make the social and physical environment more conducive for individuals to act by channeling resources (personnel, goods and services, time, money). This involves engaging networks in public and private organizations and special interest groups that control community resources in coordinative efforts to activate a broad range of interpersonal, group, and mass communication dynamics (Rogers & Storey, 1987).

The symbolic dimension is that groups with power over resources "give sanction, justification, (and) the license to act" (Rogers & Shoemaker, 1971, p. 280) influencing the rest of the community to adopt desired changes. The tangible aspect is that groups with power to allocate resources may change their internal structure (capacity) to provide opportunities for individuals to engage in behavior-change activity. These opportunities may include organizations acting as channels to reach individuals with specific behavior-change strategies; the adoption of strategies themselves by organizations; and providing a framework for individuals to influence others as volunteers working for behavior-change goals. The latter two particularly involve expanding organizational capacity in the transfer of technology, knowledge, and skills.

These views broaden the responsibility for health outcomes beyond traditional privatized relationships or the purview of traditionally defined fields. The process of community mobilization for prevention involves in part building the agenda for health and prevention through community sectors that have not heretofore possessed such an agenda. In this sense, the ideas of "health" and health outcomes have been changing to include not only the presence or absence of disease in individually centered treatment and prevention models, but, more broadly, "well being," "quality of life," and health as "community resource."

Communication is central to the entire enterprise, whether it be in affecting individuals' decisions or in affecting antecedent social and cultural conditions or public policy to make community environments supportive of healthier behaviors (Green, 1986). Research and demonstration projects alluded to earlier have provided fertile ground for understanding communication processes and effects in an overall framework of health in a more integrated fashion, especially because they make use of multiple intervention strategies operating at multiple communication levels. For example, community-based interventions such as the Minnesota Heart Health Program have used multiple health promotion and health education strategies in partnership with communities to reduce heart attacks and strokes. These have included long-term lifestyle campaigns integrating strategies including individual health counseling, class and group settings, mass and alternative media, physician and health professional education and support for developing prevention protocols in clinical practice, school-based programs, community-wide incentive and participation programs involving organizations and their members, mass screening for cardiovascular disease-related risk factors and referral to health-care personnel of those at greatest risk, promotion of available community resources for health behavior change opportunities, point-of-purchase programs, policy initiatives, and so on (Mittelmark et al., 1986).

CONCLUSION

These applied perspectives provide a much stronger bridge than has heretofore existed between the public health and medical sectors. As Green noted, the United States has adopted a national strategy of disease prevention and health promotion that includes a unified set of public health and preventive medical strategies (U.S. Surgeon General, 1979). These developments and our analysis of trends in health communication research suggest that the field's perspectives have gradually begun to expand beyond assumed institutional settings to include a more integrated consideration of effects and processes especially in community contexts. The strongest impact of these changes lies in the increasing recognition that health—like politics—is not an institution, but a set of collective behaviors that are formed and influenced through communication processes in the context of aggregate social relations and contacts (Katz, 1987). This increases the burden on health communication scholars because of the greater need to emphasize the link between varied health outcomes and varied communication processes and outcomes in community contexts. Although still in their early stages, these developments in the research agenda may go a long way toward helping to secure an "inextricable link" between health and communication, whether the nature of the link turns out to be generalizable theory or clearer articulation of complex interactions through theoretical pluralism.

REFERENCES

Allen, R. F., & Allen, J. (1987). A sense of community, a shared vision and a positive culture: core enabling factors in successful culture-based health promotion. *American Journal of Health Promotion, 2,* 40–47.

Becker, M., & Maiman, L. (1983). Models of health-related behavior. In D. Mechanic (Ed.), *Handbook of health, healthcare, and the health professions* (pp. 539–568). New York: MacMillan.

Berger, C. R., & Chaffee, S. H. (1987). The study of communication as a science. In C. R. Berger & S. H. Chaffee (Eds.), *Handbook of communication science* (pp. 15–19). Newbury Park, CA: Sage.

Blackburn, H. B. (1983). Research and demonstration projects in community cardiovascular disease prevention. *Journal of Public Health Policy, 4,* 398–421.

Bloom, S. W. (1963). The process of becoming a physician. *Annals of the American Academy, 346,* 77–87.

Blum, H. L. (1981). *Planning for health: Generics for the eighties.* New York: Human Sciences Press.

Cassata, D. M. (1978). Health communication theory and research: An overview of the communication specialist interface. In B. Ruben (Ed.), *Communication yearbook 2* (pp. 495–503). New Brunswick, NJ: Transaction-International Communication Association.

Cassata, D. M. (1980). Health communication theory and research: A definitional overview. In D. Nimmo (Ed.), *Communication yearbook 4* (pp. 583–589). New Brunswick, NJ: Transaction Books.

Chaffee, S. H. (1975). The diffusion of political information. In S. H. Chaffee (Ed.), *Political communication: issues and strategies for research* (Vol. 4, Sage Annual Reviews of Communication Research, pp. 85–128). Beverly Hills, CA: Sage.

Costello, D. E. (1977). Health communication theory and research: An overview. In B. Ruben (Ed.), *Communication yearbook 1* (pp. 557–567). New Brunswick, NJ: Transaction-International Communication Association.

Eisenstadt, S. N., & Shachar, A. (1986). *Society, culture, and urbanization.* Newbury Park, CA: Sage.

Elder, J. P., Hovell, M. F., Lasater, T. M., Wells, B. L., & Carleton, R. A. (1985). Applications of behavior modification to community health education: the case of heart disease prevention. *Health Education Quarterly, 12,* 151–168.

Fabrega, H., Jr. (1977). Perceived illness and its treatment: a naturalistic study in social medicine. *British Journal of Preventive and Social Medicine, 31,* 213–219.

Farquhar, J. W., Fortmann, S. P., Maccoby, N., Haskell, W. L., Williams, P. T., Flora, J. A., Taylor, C. B., Brown, B. W. Jr., Solomon, D. S., & Hulley, S. B. (1985). The Stanford Five-City Project: Design and Methods. *American Journal of Epidemiology, 122,* 323–334.

Finnegan, J. R., Bracht, N., & Viswanath, K. (in press). Community power and leadership analysis: formative research strategies for lifestyle campaigns. In C. T. Salmon (Ed.), *Information campaigns: Balancing social values and social marketing* (Vol. 18, Sage Annual Reviews of Communication Research). Newbury Park, CA: Sage.

Green, L. W. (1984). Health education models. In J. D. Matarazzo, S. M. Weiss, J. A. Herd, N. E. Miller, S. M. Weiss (Eds.), *Behavioral health: A handbook of health enhancement and disease prevention* (pp. 181–197). New York: Wiley.

Green, L. W. (1986). Prevention and health education. In J. M. Last (Ed.), *Public health and preventive medicine* (12 ed., pp. 1089–1106). New York: Appleton-Century-Crofts.

Halloran, J. D. (1981). The context of mass communications research. In E. McAnany, J. Schnitman, & N. Janus (Eds.), *Communication and social change* (pp. 21–57). New York: Praeger.

Janz, N. K., & Becker, M. H. (1984). The health belief model: A decade later. *Health Education Quarterly, 11,* 1–47.

Katz, E. (1987). Communication research since Lazarsfeld. *Public Opinion Quarterly, 51,* S25–S45.

Keys, A. (1980). *The seven countries study.* Cambridge, MA: Harvard University Press.

Kreps, G. (1988). The pervasive role of information in health and health care: Implications for health communication policy. In J. A. Anderson (Ed.), *Communication yearbook 11* (pp. 238–276). Newbury Park, CA: Sage.

Kreps, G. L., & Thornton, B. C. (1984). *Health communication.* White Plains, NY: Longman.

Langlie, J. K. (1977). Social networks, health beliefs, and preventive health behavior. *Journal of Health and Social Behavior, 18,* 244–260.

Mittelmark, M., Luepker, R. V., Jacobs, D., Bracht, N., Carlaw, R., Crow, R., Finnegan, J. R., Grimm, R. H., Jeffery, R. W., Kline, F. G., Mullis, R. M., Murray, D. M., Pechacek, T., Perry, C. P., Pirie, P. L., & Blackburn, H. B. (1986). Community-wide prevention of cardiovascular disease: Education strategies of the Minnesota Heart Health Program. *Preventive Medicine, 15,* 1–17.

Parsons, T. (1951). *The social system.* Glencoe, IL: The Free Press.

Pettegrew, L. S. (1988). Theoretical plurality in health communication. In J. A. Anderson (Ed.), *Communication yearbook 11* (pp. 298–308). Newbury Park, CA: Sage.

Reardon, K. K. (1988). The role of persuasion in health promotion and disease prevention: Review and commentary. In J. A. Anderson (Ed.), *Communication yearbook 11,* (pp. 277–297). Newbury Park, CA: Sage.

Robbins, A. (1985). Public health in the next decade. *Journal of Public Health Policy, 6,* 440–446.

Rogers, E. M., & Shoemaker, F. F. (1971). *Communication of innovations: A cross-cultural approach* (2nd ed.). New York: The Free Press.

Rogers, E. M., & Storey, J. D. (1987). Communication campaigns. In C. R. Berger & S. H. Chaffee (Eds.), *Handbook of communication science* (pp. 817–846). Newbury Park: Sage.

Somers, A. R., & Weisfeld, V. D. (1986). Individual behavior and health. In J. M. Last (Ed.), *Public health and preventive medicine* (12 ed., pp. 983–997). New York: Appleton-Century-Crofts.

Starr, P. (1982). *The social transformation of American medicine.* New York: Basic Books.

Suchman, E. A. (1966). Health orientation and medical care. *American Journal of Public Health, 56,* 97–105.

Suchman, E. A. (1967). Preventive health behavior: A model for research on community health campaigns. *Journal of Health and Social Behavior, 8,* 197–209.

Terris, M. (1986). Editorial: What is health promotion? *Journal of Public Health Policy, 7,* 147–151.

U.S. Surgeon General. (1979). *Healthy people: The Surgeon General's report on health and disease prevention.* Washington: U.S. Department of Health, Education and Welfare.

II

HEALTH COMMUNICATION WITHIN MEDICAL CONTEXTS: INTERPERSONAL, SMALL GROUP, AND ORGANIZATIONAL ISSUES

3

Patient Health Care:
Issues in Interpersonal Communication

Teresa L. Thompson
University of Dayton

The interpersonal communication occurring between the providers and receivers of health care has been a focus of dissatisfaction for both dyad members for some time (e.g., Bird, 1955). As a result, the communication characterizing this dyad has also been a topic of considerable research. The research has been conducted by medical professionals as well as by investigators in most of the social sciences. Because a variety of disciplines have been represented, many of the researchers have been unaware of other research relevant to their own and have not incorporated or built upon the foundation provided by this other research. Because one of the bases of science is the cumulative development of knowledge (Kaplan, 1964), research that does not build upon previous information results in much duplication of effort and slows the scientific process. An overview of health communication research indicates that much of the available corpus does, indeed, ignore earlier research on similar concerns published in other disciplines (Thompson, 1984). Therefore, this chapter integrates and synthesizes this literature to provide a basis upon which future researchers may build.

Communication between the provider and the patient is crucial not only to patient satisfaction with the health professional, but also to the health-care delivery process itself (Dance, 1970; Levy, 1985; Lochman, 1983). Effective message sending is necessary for both (a) patient communication of symptoms and physical problems, and (b) physician communication of instructions. Additionally, the relationship between a patient and a health-care professional is created through the communication that occurs between them. This influences their degree of under-standing of each other and the openness of their communication. Open-ness and trust are important variables when communicating about the taboo topics that may be necessary components of health professional–patient discussions (Meize-Grochowski, 1984). Lucas (1985) found that even a reciprocal exchange of background information during the ini-tial interview improved physician–patient rapport.

The purpose of this chapter is to summarize and synthesize research in this important area. The focus of the review is on interpersonal communication between providers and receivers of health care and, to a lesser degree, on communication among health-care providers. Most of the research on communication among health providers is discussed in the chapters on small group and organizational communication. The reader will note that little of the research presented herein actually takes the systemic perspective, even though the health-care context was the model originally envisioned by Parsons (1951) in *The Social System*. Much of the research, however, does consider the interdepen-dence of the participants and looks at how one member's behavior affects the other. Several other important systems concepts are also represented in the research. These include: (a) feedback and control, the foundations of a cybernetic systems perspective; (b) equivocality or uncertainty reduction; (c) homeostasis; and (d) inputs–throughputs–outputs. Basically, the provider–patient interaction should be seen as an equifinal cybernetic system with a goal of improved health. Commu-nication can function as an input or throughput to amplify or counteract deviation toward that goal.

General Observations

The research that has been conducted on health communication has been much less systematic than is generally seen as desirable in the social sciences. One symptom of this is the lack of accumulation of knowledge, as was previously mentioned. Another example may be found in the methods used in this research area. Although it is fre-quently fruitful to rely upon a variety of methods to increase validity, research that is ignorant of previous knowledge may become method-ologically haphazard. Because the researchers all start from scratch, they begin at a descriptive/observational level. This would be appro-priate if they were not *all* doing it. As a result of this, more sophisticated methods that are appropriate for the examination of specific, causal relationships are underused.

The research has been divided into several content areas for the purposes of review. Our review is representative rather than comprehensive. The following areas are discussed: (a) physician–patient communication, focusing specifically on satisfaction, control, interviewing, and compliance with health instructions; (b) nurse–patient communication; and (c) the neglected health professions.

Overall, a recurring theme is present throughout all of this research: There is a need for increased communication in the health professions and for more sensitivity to communication. Consistent with this is the suggestion of metacommunication—talking about how we communicate (Elder, 1963). If the notion of a physician saying, "Well, what I hear you saying is . . ." or "Let me paraphrase what I think you're saying . . ." sounds unlikely to you, you may appreciate the difficulty of addressing this research area.

PHYSICIAN–PATIENT COMMUNICATION

Historians identify two basic assumptions of modern medicine: germ theory and preventive medicine (Wain, 1970). Each leads to a different emphasis within the doctor–patient interaction. During the middle ages and for a time beyond, it was assumed that each disease manifested itself in different symptoms in different patients. It was, therefore, the responsibility of the patient to tell the physician what was wrong. With the development of germ theory this assumption was discarded, and responsibility went to the physician to diagnose the ailment. This, thus, placed the emphasis on the health-care provider. When the notion of preventive medicine developed more recently, the emphasis shifted back to the patient, who is supposed to take greater responsibility for his or her own health. Most of the research that follows still places emphasis on the care provider, despite current trends that might argue against this.

Satisfaction

In an analysis of doctor–patient interaction based on representation in art, Swiderski (1976) concluded that, "the pictures show the physician's mastery and the patient's comfort in that mastery. They make disease into visual knowledge that is open and shared, and suggest that disease is finite" (p. 5). Although this may be the view people have shared in the past, or the view we would like to have, much empirical research questions its current applicability. Research indicates that patients are satisfied with the medical care they receive from doctors, but are dissatisfied with the communication accompanying that care (Decastro, 1972; Fuller & Quesada, 1973; Skipper, 1965a). Because some physicians see a concern with "bedside manner" as a concession to "selling" medicine (Korsch & Negrete, 1972), these problems may not be easy to overcome.

Several communicative behaviors have been identified that influence the patient's satisfaction with communication. The amount of warmth and friendliness shown by the doctor is positively related to satisfaction (Daly & Hulka, 1975; Korsch, Gozzi, & Francis, 1968). Korsch and Negrete (1972), based on observations of 800 doctor–patient interactions, found that (a) less than 5% of doctor's communication was personal or friendly, (b) most doctor's self-reports indicated they thought they were behaving in a friendly manner, and (c) physicians were much friendlier to children than to adults. Similarly, Street and Wiemann's (1987) study found that "patients' satisfaction with medical care was positively related to degree of the physician's perceived interpersonal involvement and expressiveness and negatively associated with perceived communicative dominance" (p. 605). And Matthews, Sledge, and Lieberman's (1987) study concluded that interpersonal skills are valued just as much by patients as are traditional clinical skills.

In perhaps the most thorough examination of the factors related to patients' satisfaction with medical care, Lochman (1983) determined relationships between satisfaction and the communicative behaviors of clarity and retention of physician's communication to patients, physicians' affiliative behavior, and physician's control. Several other noncommunicative behaviors were also related to satisfaction.

Dreyfuss (1986) cited findings by Frankel and Beckman indicating some specific communicative behaviors that may lead to satisfaction: interrupting and listening. Frankel and Beckman found that patients described their complaints for an average of only 18 seconds before being interrupted. Only 23% of the patients were able to tell the doctor everything they had planned to mention.

Lack of communication with the patient or the patient's family is another frequently cited problem (Crown, 1971; Schwartz & Overton, 1987), particularly because patients have a desire for information but do not demand it (Adler, 1977). Even cancer patients report that high uncertainty and anxiety can be addressed by communication (Molleman et al., 1984). Patients who do ask direct, rather than indirect, questions also demonstrate more satisfaction with the medical interaction (Roter, 1984).

Important contexts requiring more communication include clear explanations of the nature and cause of the illness (Korsch et al., 1968; Skipper, 1965b), the treatment that was prescribed (Decastro, 1972), and the expected duration of the illness (Decastro, 1972). The importance of the return visit is also inadequately discussed (Decastro, 1972).

Aasterud (1965) concluded that explanations are particularly important prior to operations. She found that appropriate detail of the explanation was an important variable. For example, anxious patients should be given more detail about medical procedures, although patients who appear calm and unconcerned prior to the operation are frequently angry after it if they have not been given an adequate explanation of the procedure. Timing of the explanation is another concern for doctors. Aasterud concluded that an explanation should occur substantially in advance of the operation if it will necessitate major changes in the patient's lifestyle, and shortly prior to the operation if only minor adaptation is required. Explanations after the procedure are better than none at all, but her guideline is: Do not surprise the patient. Meyers' (1965) research reached a similar conclusion, but also found that irrelevant communication when a patient needed an explanation was worse than no communication at all. Explanations are particularly necessary during unusual procedures, such as an initial pelvic exam (Broadmore, Carr-Gregg, & Hutton, 1986).

In addition to the need for explanations, patient satisfaction with communication is influenced by the physician's awareness of the patient's concerns (Daly & Hulka, 1975; Korsch et al., 1968). Liptak, Hulka, and Cassel (1977) further found that a doctor's awareness of a mother's concerns about her child is positively related to mother–child adaptation, and that physician communication is positively related to maternal satisfaction with medical care. Mothers are concerned about their physician's disregard of remarks they make about things they think are important (Korsch & Negrete, 1972). Of these mothers, however, 26% did not even mention their greatest concern to the doctor because of lack of opportunity or encouragement (Daly & Hulka, 1975; Korsch & Negrete, 1972). Arntson, Droge, and Fassi (1978) also found that patients do not ask for explanations. Even when information that is relevant is given by the patient's family, it is frequently ignored by the physician (Crown, 1971).

Further patient dissatisfaction with communication is based on the physician's use of technical language or jargon (Daly & Hulka, 1975), which mystifies the patient. This appears to occur in 50% of all cases (Korsch & Negrete, 1972). Although reliance on medical language may be necessary to communicate some ideas, most patients will not understand it (Samora, Saunders, & Larson, 1961). This leads to a lack of comprehension of information in the patients, most of whom are reluctant to raise questions (Korsch & Negrete, 1972). Korsch, Freeman, and Negrete (1971) suggest that the physician needs to speak the patient's language, because the patient is certainly not able to speak the physician's language.

In a provocative examination of medical language from a general semantics perspective, Baziak and Denton (1960) extended this line of analysis past the realm of misunderstanding to argue that medical personnel perceive only certain aspects of the patient. These aspects are determined by cultural and linguistic preconditioning. Doctors label patients as "symptoms" and give patients and nurses "orders." Patients are labeled as "not cooperative" and are communicated with according to the perception that patients "complain." The emphasis on the medical terminology causes medical personnel to perceive only those aspects of the patient. This, of course, is deviation-amplifying in a cybernetic sense, as care providers get farther and farther away from seeing the whole patient.

Raimbault, Cachin, Limal, Eliacheff, and Rappaport (1975), in an analysis of medical discourse, found that doctors evade emotional issues in favor of quasi-scientific expressions that are not understood by patients. Moreover, physicians frequently talk at cross-purposes with patients and their families, ignoring issues raised by the patient. Toombs (1987) concurred that physicians and patients encounter the experience from different worlds of meaning.

Other barriers to doctor–patient communication include patients' reluctance to initiate communication because of awe, fear of negative reactions, suspicions that they will not receive good answers anyway, the small amount of time patients have with doctors, the patients' perceptions that doctors and nurses are overworked and have little time (all from Skipper, 1965a, 1965b) and cultural and class differences between the doctor and the patient (Samora et al., 1961; Walker, 1973). Suggestions to overcome these problems include increased emphasis on nonverbal sensitivity in the doctor, because the patient may be unwilling or unable to verbally communicate the problem (Friedman, 1979). This becomes even more important when it is realized that up to 50% of the physician's time spent in patient care, especially in general practice, pediatrics, and internal medicine, is spent on problems that are primarily psychological and involve a need for understanding and communication (Korsch & Negrete, 1972).

Kupst, Dresser, Schulman, and Paul (1975) compared four methods of physician communication—a single communication, both written and oral communication, physician repetition, and patient restatement—and found that patient restatement increased retention of information, but no significant differences were discovered with anxiety or satisfaction as the dependent variables. Focusing on a different set of variables, Egbert, Battit, Wilch, and Bartlett (1964) found that preoperative encouragement and education by anesthesiologists reduced postoperative pain and resulted in earlier dismissal from the hospital.

Heszen-Klemens and Lapinska (1984) reported one of the most thorough and interesting studies of the interrelationships between physician–patient interaction and treatment effectiveness. They determined that doctors' directiveness, doctors' emotional attitude toward the patient, and patient partnership status (system inputs) had effects on patients' health (system output). Apparently, these behaviors affect both compliance with instructions and the likelihood of patients' spontaneous (extraneous) health activity (system throughputs).

This last finding is consistent with work conducted by Pruyn, Ruckman, van Brunschot, and van de Borne (1985). Their examination of breast cancer patients indicated that those patients who believed they had received insufficient and unclear information from their physicians were more likely to adopt an unproven diet remedy. Although the use of the diet is not cause for concern, there is a fear that patients will stop normal treatment and rely exclusively on the unproven diet. The role of communication in this process is emphasized by the finding of Ben-Sira (1980) that a lack of emotional involvement and support by physicians lessens patients' confidence in regular treatment and in the physicians themselves. Such patients are more likely to try their own alternatives.

Most of the research reported here has focused on patient dissatisfaction with the doctor–patient interaction and on behavior that the physician should change. Other research has examined the physician's dissatisfaction with the interaction with the patient. For instance, patient listening ability and recall of instructions (Ray & Bostrom, 1987) and unmet dependency needs (Powers, 1985) may be concerns.

Additionally, both the physician and the patient frequently find their expectations about the encounter unfulfilled (Fuller & Quesada, 1973; Reader, Pratt, & Mudd, 1957; Walker, 1973) and need to communicate those expectations and provide feedback. Fuller and Quesada described a deviation amplifying "spiralling down," which occurs when one person's expectations are not met, causing that person to become unwilling or unable to hear or meet the needs of the other. Each, experiencing greater frustration and distrust, becomes less attentive to the wishes or needs of the other and filters out increasingly unacceptable demands while trying to get his or her own needs met. Physicians are not unwilling to show impatience or irritation with patients (Korsch & Negrete, 1972). This process means, of course, that the physician's needs may also be unmet. Fuller and Quesada suggest that deviation counteracting or "spiralling up" may occur if either member of the dyad tries to hear what is positive in the other's communication and emphasize this. This may return the system to a homeostatic state.

The research on satisfaction has, thus, indicated several important things. Although there is much satisfaction with medical care, there is also quite a bit of dissatisfaction on the part of both patients and health-care providers. Most of the dissatisfaction for the patient relates to communication variables. Providing more detailed explanations with less use of jargon decreases this dissatisfaction, as does sharing control.

Control

In the process of their discussion of spiralling, Fuller and Quesada (1973) described a control struggle in physician–patient interaction. The notion of control is an important one for an understanding of the health-care system from a cybernetic perspective. This concern is also implicit in Walker's (1973) suggestion of the importance of authority in physician–patient interaction and in Neal's (1962) observations that patients are likely to demand control. Although Friedman and DiMatteo (1979) argue that the patient should be treated as a consumer rather than an object and should be given more responsibility and control, the data indicate that physicians control interactions (Coulthard & Ashby, 1975; Korsch & Negrete, 1972) and are dissatisfied by patient attempts to assert control (Ort, Ford, & Liske, 1964). Observations of doctor–patient communication demonstrate physician initiation of information exchanges and control of timing, a lack of response to patient initiation attempts, interruption of patients, the asking of leading questions (Coulthard & Ashby, 1975), physician monopolization of talk time and the raising of fears but failure to address them (Korsch & Negrete, 1972). Physicians ask twice as many questions and give twice as many commands as patients (Arntson et al., 1978). Neal (1962) reported that doctors are threatened by patient control attempts, although a more successful outcome results when the patient is active rather than passive and harsh treatment or scaring leads to a poor outcome (Korsch & Negrete, 1972; Tryon & Leonard, 1965).

Other research on control has pointed out that perceived control by the patient will affect health outcomes (Brenders, 1986). And Barnard (1985) argued that changes in shared control during the physician–patient interaction can occur only with reform of the ordinary pragmatic structures in everyday practice as it is currently conducted.

This difficulty in sharing control is confirmed by O'Hair's (1989) analysis of videotaped physician–patient interactions. The predominant transaction mode discovered in these data was competitive symmetry, in which the two participants vie for control (a one-up statement responded to with a one-up statement). Second most common was complementarity, with patients twice as willing as physicians to yield control after it was sought by the physicians (a one-up followed by a one-down). Physicians were also twice as willing to assume control of the exchange after it was offered by patients (a one-down followed by a one-up). Patients were more likely to respond to a one-down message with their own one-down message than were doctors. Following a one-across message, physicians generally responded with one-up control maneuvers, whereas patients rarely did. Generally, however, "patients were not particularly submissive when control of the exchange was attempted by the physician" (O'Hair, 1989, p. 109).

A related study also looked at the interrelationships between physician and patient communicative behavior. Ferguson (1987) concluded that: (a) when the physician asks more questions, the patient asks fewer questions; (b) discussion of nonmedical topics leads to more shared communication; and (c) physicians who quiz patients typically interrupt the patients to do so. She also found some sex differences, in that female physicians received significantly more patient questions and spent more time explaining.

We have seen that control struggles are frequent in health-care interactions. Most health-care providers control these interactions, but some patients attempt to assert control, as well. A more effective outcome results when control is shared than when it is monopolized by one person.

Other Sources of Dissatisfaction

In addition to dissatisfaction regarding control, doctors also tend to be dissatisfied with patient's lack of compliance with instructions (Korsch & Negrete, 1972) and report that a frequent problem is overcoming the patient's own diagnosis (Coulthard & Ashby, 1975) or convincing the patient that his or her spouse's diagnosis is wrong (Walker, 1973). Empirical study indicates listening problems on the part of patients, as well. They frequently report that physicians have not told them things that in actuality have been recorded on tape (Korsch & Negrete, 1972). Samora et al. (1961) also found that patients may be unwilling to hear unpleasant news and that poor memory can add to these problems. Carnerie (1987) echoed these concerns.

The theme of most of this research, however, is that these problems may be solved with more and better communication and communication training (e.g., Nutting, 1986). Most agree with Frank Dance (1970): "the quality of communication seriously affected the degree of medical success" (p. 30). Although communication can be time consuming and physicians may believe this will cause them to make less money (Walker, 1973), empirical evidence indicates that, in the longest physician–patient sessions, most time is consumed by a failure to communicate (Korsch & Negrete, 1972). These authors also conclude that neglect of communication may account for the flourishing business of quacks and faith healers, who provide the emotional reassurance lacking in physician–patient encounters. Simoni and Ball (1975) provide data supporting this hypothesis. They found that, among the poor, medical hucksters rank higher in credibility, honesty, usefulness, and helpfulness than medical personnel, who are far down the list. Hoffmann (1988) made a similar contention regarding the role of play acting in medicine as he wrote of "The Doctor as Dramatist."

Interviewing

The initial doctor–patient interview is an important data-gathering and relationship-building tool and has been examined by several researchers. Helfer and Ealy (1972), in a 3-year study of medical students' interviewing skills, found a need for interviewing training among seniors in medical school. Kline and Ceropski (1985) also reported that communication skills deteriorate during medical school. Because less than 10% of doctors do a good job of even history taking in the interview (Mace, 1971), and the more difficult skills of empathy and clarification are positively related to accuracy of diagnoses (Marks, Goldberg, & Hillier, 1979), Kline and Ceropski (1985) identified several effective interviewing strategies. These include listening carefully, reassuring, showing empathy, verbally inviting expressions of the patient's concerns, discussing assumptions, and nonpossessive warmth and genuineness. Kline and Ceropski (1985) also investigated some of the skills related to effective interviewing. They advocated communication strategies adapted to the specific patient and found that the propensity to do this was related to medical students' ability to construe dispositional and motivational characteristics of the patients.

Engel (1973) added recording, relating, and overcoming uneasiness to the list of important interviewing skills. In his classic treatise, Bird (1955) was even more specific about these skills. He encouraged doctors to allow enough time for the interview, conduct it in a quiet, uninterrupted spot, show interest in the patient, look for signs of distress, continue talking throughout the exam but listen more than talk, not diagnose in the interview, let information sink in, not become involved in arguments with the patient, avoid writing as much as possible, look for patterns in the patient's family or behavior, ask open questions, be precise in terminology, take nothing for granted, question assumptions, and try to find the real issue behind anxiety. In appropriate contexts, the physician is exhorted to meet the patient's anger head-on or bring hidden anger out into the open.

In some of the few studies truly beginning from a systemic view, Hawes reported several observations of communication patterns in doctor–patient interviews. He found that interviewers establish similar patterns with different interviewees (Hawes, 1972a). In further analyses of these data, he looked at differences between directive and nondirective interviews (Hawes, 1972b). He concluded that directive interviews include more clarification and elaboration, while in nondirective interviews more asking and answering of specific questions is observed. And, Hawes (1973) reported that clarification and questioning reduce uncertainty or equivocality, whereas negative reinforcement, generalizing, and quiet increase uncertainty. Questions function as initiators of communication cycles or patterns.

The research thus indicates numerous communication skills that can be developed by health-care providers to make the health interview a more effective data-gathering and relational-development tool. Adaptation, clarification, and questioning seem to be among these. Other skills will certainly be identified that relate to effective physician–patient communication and interviewing. Regardless, the effectiveness of this communication will influence the patient's compliance with the doctor's instructions (Lane, 1983).

Compliance

Compliance is, of course, basically a cybernetic control notion. The health-care provider is using feedback to the patient to regulate the patient's behavior. Research indicates a low rate of compliance with doctor's orders (Dervin, Harlock, Atwood, & Garzona, 1980). Noncompliance has been reported to average around 50% (Miller, 1975). This lack of compliance creates health hazards and leads to a waste of resources and frustration on the part of the doctor (Stone, 1979). Some noncommunication variables influence compliance, because adherence increases with status of the message source (Levine, Moss, Ramsey, & Fleishman, 1978) and when patient expectations are met (Francis, Korsch, & Morris, 1969); adherence to physician instructions decreases when they necessitate a major change in habits or lifestyle (Charney, 1972). Patient satisfaction also increases compliance (Francis et al., 1969).

The communicative behaviors of simplicity and specificity of instructions (Charney, 1972; Korsch & Negrete, 1972), physician expressions of trust in the mother's caretaking and offers of continued interest in the child (Korsch & Negrete, 1972), provisions of explanations and demonstrations of warmth (Francis et al., 1969), and rapport building (DiMatteo, 1979) also appear to result in adherence to instructions. A lack of compliance is associated with formality, antagonism, and mutual withholding of information (Davis, 1968). In particular, Davis found that, when physicians seek information without giving feedback to the patient, noncompliance increases. Tension-relieving behaviors such as joking also increase compliance (Davis, 1971). Compliance can frequently be hurt by unclear instructions, such as "cut down on starches." Most patients do not have accurate information about what foods do and do not contain starch (Ley & Spelman, 1967).

Some strategies have been identified that are used to increase adherence in patients. All of these strategies examine cybernetic feedback mechanisms used to counteract deviation. In a review of this research, Lane (1983) found that doctors typically try the following approaches: (a) give the patient a thorough explanation; (b) tell him or her the benefits of the advice; (c) get tough; and (d) withdraw. If noncompliance still results, physicians: (a) overwhelm the patient with knowledge; (b) tell the patient of the dire consequences that will occur if he or she does not comply; (c) disclose to patients; or (d) use personal persuasion tactics.

Rodin and Janis (1979) provide evidence indicating that this last strategy may be the most effective one. In a study of the bases of power most useful for obtaining compliance, they discovered that referent power was preferred. Referent power can be built by the physician's emphasis on similarities between him or herself and the patient, demonstration of a benevolent, unselfish attitude and the provision of acceptance statements to the patient. This should be followed by occasional contact with the patient to reinforce the building of self-esteem (Rodin & Janis, 1979).

Other evidence suggests that medical professionals may have difficulty demonstrating these behaviors because they are unable to identify them. Lane (1983) found that health-care workers were not able to discriminate between instructing and caring communications.

Burgoon and his colleagues (Burgoon, Birk et al., 1987; Burgoon, Parrott et al., 1987) have studied the compliance problem by using an application of persuasion/communication theory from other settings and a motivational perspective. They focused on the use of verbally aggressive strategies in their two-part study. Their conclusions indicated that physicians perceive themselves as using expertise more frequently than verbal aggression, and use verbally aggressive compliance-gaining strategies only with patients with severe illnesses and a history of noncompliance. The physicians feel that they use verbally aggressive strategies more frequently in initial interactions. Patients, however, see these physicians as using verbally unaggressive strategies during initial interactions. Although less-aggressive strategies had a positive effect on patient satisfaction, more aggressive ones did not have a strong negative impact.

Finally, Conrad (1985) argued that we can improve compliance only by looking at the *meaning* of medication to the patient. He claimed that "What appears to be noncompliance from a medical perspective may actually be a form of asserting control over one's disorder" (p. 29). Implicit in Conrad's argument is a perspective on compliance more consistent with the transactional nature of communication than is found in much of the other research cited herein. Most of the research has focused on compliance as a one-way communicative act—the care provider communicates a message and the patient receives and responds to the message. This perspective ignores the transactional (rather than actional) nature of the communication process.

Regardless of this limitation, the research conducted to date does provide some helpful information to health-care providers. Rather than being basically a "personality" problem, compliance can be conceptualized as a communicative issue. Compliance or cooperation can be improved by sharing control with patients, by seeking feedback, by giving unambiguous information and by demonstrating warmth and concern.

Although the research just reported has focused on physicians, much of it also applies to nurse–patient communication. The research discussed in the next section, however, focuses specifically on this process.

NURSE–PATIENT COMMUNICATION

The role of the nurse in health communication bears both similarities and dissimilarities to that of the physician. Skipper (1965b) argued that the nurse is in a pivotal position on the patient–care team. His or her coursework has emphasized social relations more than any other health-care team member. Despite this, evidence shows tendencies toward depersonalizing the patient. Although nurses claim that patients should be treated as people rather than cases, they do not communicate as they profess they should nor as they think they do (Skipper, 1965b).

Tarasuk, Rhymes, and Leonard (1965) argued that communication skills are as important as any other skills in the helping professions, including technical competence. Their experiment found that patients experience relief from pain more quickly, thoroughly, and without the use of drugs if nurses approach them extending support and recognition and explore individual patients rather than rely on assumptions. Other research has indicated that postoperative vomiting can be reduced by preoperative communication between nurse and patient that helps prepare the patient for the experience (Dumas, Anderson, & Leonard, 1965). And Dodge (1965) found that a nurse's willingness to keep patients informed is related to the nurse's feelings of adequacy. Nurses who feel less confident about their skills are less willing to communicate with patients because they are afraid of exposing their own inadequacies.

One way to improve communication, then, could be based on building nurses' skills and confidence. Aguilera (1967) demonstrated that communication can also be improved through training nurses to touch patients more. When nurses are encouraged to increase touch, the amount of verbal interaction and rapport between caregivers and patients also increases. Nurses are more likely to approach patients. These improvements appear after about 8 days of instruction, are more pronounced on the evening than the day shift, and show no sex differences. Touch, then, is a systemic throughput leading to positive outputs.

Other attempts to improve nurse–patient communication and health care have focused on such variables as manipulation and caring. Hughes (1980), for instance, argued that a *compulsion* to care can become destructive and manipulative; Kitson (1987) concurred that a definition of care must be understood and argued that a lay view of caring may be more productive than a traditional nursing definition.

Kalisch (1971) has attempted to improve nurse–patient communication through training nurses in empathy. The program involved role playing, role models, and experiential and didactic training. Improvement was shown on a paper-and-pencil measure and self- and instructor evaluations, but not on patient evaluations or a measure of predictive empathy. The improvement that was observed had persisted in a later follow-up.

One of the more innovative attempts to improve hospital staff–patient communication entailed "graffiti therapy" (Shulman, Peven, & Byrne, 1973). The walls of a mental health unit were lined with paper and everyone was encouraged to write on it. Shulman et al. found that this opened up lines of communication, as the patients and staff wrote notes to each other, and provided the staff with insight about communicating with patients.

Many of the other suggestions for improvement of nurse–patient communication have been based simply on basic communication principles. Going beyond this is an interesting piece of research titled, "What is the patient saying?" (Elder, 1963). Because research has indicated that nurses frequently make hasty and inaccurate judgments about patients' messages (Tarasuk et al., 1965) and patients do not consistently communicate needs well (Elder, 1963), the nurse needs to be aware that, from a systemic view, communication occurs on content, relationship, and identity levels (Villard & Whipple, 1974). Any message communicates information not only about the content, but about the patient and the relationship between the patient and the health professional. Elder argued that the behavior initially shown by patients is not necessarily a good index of their discomfiture. Frequently, patients do not realize what is making them uncomfortable, and the stress they are experiencing may inhibit expression and make feedback difficult. Elder reported an observational study that indicated that patients often need to communicate about emotional issues to get them off their chests before physical problems can be addressed. Another pattern necessitated administering to patient's physical needs before the issue of real concern to them, an emotional one, could be discussed.

The type of communication that Elder described is difficult, she suggested, because nurses are not rewarded for communicating with patients; the emphasis is on getting as much work done as possible. However, when the nurses do have more time, they do not use it to communicate with patients (Aydelotte, 1960; New, Nite, & Callahan, 1959).

One of the more interesting studies of nurse–patient communication was a participant observation investigation of reassurance. Gregg (1965) found that the reassurance provided by nurses frequently communicates to patients "your feelings are unimportant." Reassurance can be disconfirming, if it does not address the concern that the patient is trying to communicate. Telling the patient that there is nothing to worry about prior to an operation does not calm or reassure him or her, while listening to feelings and providing information can reassure. Gregg observed that the mere presence of another person can be reassuring to some patients. False reassurance or distraction, however, does not work.

In a related study, Buchsbaum (1986) argued that the goals of reassurance should include not only relieving the patient's anxiety, but also restoring his or her sense of autonomy. Buchsbaum emphasized that successful reassurance rests more on communicative ability than on understanding of human pathology.

The communicative role of the nurse is, thus, an important one. Nurses are frequently in greater contact with patients than are physicians. The communication between nurses and patients influences recovery and amount of pain. Nurses are also important in providing reassurance.

Communication with Other Staff Members

Other research on nurses has focused on the nurse–adolescent relationship (Long, 1985; Rubin, 1986), disclosure practices (Trandel-Korenchuk, 1987), and nurses' communicative effectiveness (Willmington &

Willmington, 1988). This research has all been primarily concerned with the patient and does not have the welfare of the nurse as its focus. Additional research has examined the stress and conflict experienced by this professional. Morse and Piland (1981) reported difficulties for nurses when communicating with peers and physicians. Doctor–nurse communication tends to be one way, with nurses allowed little feedback. This allows little opportunity to counteract deviation. This is consistent with the findings of Cunningham and Wilcox (1984) in their study of the bind produced when a doctor gives a nurse a harmful order. Morse and Piland also found that communication with other nurses requires even more communication skills than communicating with physicians or patients! Redland (1983) expressed similar concerns, as did Worobey and Cummings (1984). They discussed difficulties in the nurse–administrator relationship requiring special emphasis on skills such as listening, addressing, persuading, and managing conflicts.

Malone, Berkowitz, and Klein (1962) found role conflict for nurses because they are expected to care for patients, educate them, *and* administer the unit. They have neither the time nor the resources to do all of these. And Albrecht (1982) examined nurses' methods of handling the stress that is unavoidable in this position. She found that the most effective strategies were prayer, talking with friends and family outside the hospital, and talking with others in different units within the hospital. Withdrawal and drinking are not effective, but seeking support from one's supervisor can be. More recent research on support has been discussed in Albrecht and Adelman (1987). The importance of trust in nurse–nurse interaction has also been discussed (Northouse, 1979).

The Neglected Health Professions

Two other important health professions have each been addressed by a small amount of research—dentistry and physical therapy. Although dentists constitute the second largest group of primary, direct service health professionals in the country (Young & Smith, 1972), the research on communication of relevance to dentists has been especially limited. What is available seems to be composed, for the most part, of suggestions about areas of awareness that dental professionals should cultivate. Kreps (1981) and Plainfield (1969) advocate attention to nonverbal details because of their influence on the patient. Other researchers caution dentists about language. The dental student spends his or her academic career learning to speak a specialized language that decreases the ability to share meaning with patients (Vowles, 1970). In particular, dentists need to realize the meanings that patients may have for words

(Spaan, 1964) and should avoid words that suggest to the patient pain or anxiety (Jan, 1964). Dangott, Thornton, and Page (1978) investigated the communication surrounding pain in more detail. They found that dentists tend to be disconfirming when patients express or experience pain. Most dentists deny pain and many claim that patients "think they are going to have pain so some of them actually feel pain when they do not have any" (Dangott et al., 1978, p. 33). Even those dentists who do not deny the pain do not show concern for the patient's experience.

The final health profession to have benefited from some study of communication is physical therapy. Most of the interest in this field appears to be on the communication of information among physical therapists, and simply bemoans the poor writing skills of members of the profession (e.g., Special Communication, *Physical Therapy*, 1977).

Many other pieces directed toward physical therapists are "how-to" articles: how to interview patients (Croft, 1980); how to answer questions (Rochelle, 1966); how to give a speech (Sanger, 1964); or how to gain patient compliance (Mayo, 1978). This last article relies almost exclusively on the compliance literature reported earlier, but applies the principles and recommendations to physical therapists. Only one piece of empirical research was found pertaining to communication and physical therapy. Rubin, Judd, and Conine (1977) report an experiment designed to increase empathy through a training program. The results indicated that empathy could be improved and retained, at least through an eighteen month followup. The physical therapy students in the control group were unable to recognize an empathic response, and could not initiate empathic communication (Rubin et al., 1977).

There are obviously many other areas relevant to all of the professions discussed to this point that require the attention of health communication researchers. Additionally, although we may be able to generalize much of the research on the health professions that have been studied to the other health fields, that generalizability must be empirically determined. Many of the health areas listed earlier have not been the subject of *any* communication research. Of particular interest may be the pharmacist. He or she is more accessible to the typical patient than are most other health professionals. One has only to walk to the corner drugstore to see a pharmacist. It is likely that he or she can have a great impact on variables such as the patient's compliance with drug-related instructions. Investigation into pharmacist–patient communication is an open and potentially fruitful region. Other professions that may prove fruitful for researchers include med techs, social workers, and dieticians, who also play an important role in the compliance process (Thompson, 1986).

CONCLUSIONS

The research cited herein spans approximately 30 years. Although we now know considerably more about the interpersonal context of health care than we used to, more questions remain. Of current concern is the impact that communication processes have on legal action taken by patients against physicians. Recent research by May (1985) concluded that communication problems alone are not responsible for legal actions taken by dissatisfied patients, but

> when the resolution of a dispute involves going to a lawyer, patients have experienced compounded complaints including (a) professional failure in treatment, (b) a lack of communication by the doctor about the nature of diagnosis and (c) some form of insensitivity from the doctor that has been morally upsetting to them. (p. 31)

Because insensitivity must be communicated before it is known, two of these three components can only be resolved through communication. The research implications of this issue are strong. This message was also echoed by Davison (1985), in his keynote address to the Summer Conference on Health Communication: "conflicts that develop in the course of medical decision-making are not strictly of an ethical nature, but are due simply to a failure in communication between the parties involved" (p. 3).

One focus not yet taken by health communication researchers is an examination of the impact of various traditions of health care (allopathic, homeopathic, naturopathic, etc.; cf. Logan & Hunt, 1978; Moore, Van Arsdale, Glittenberg, & Aldrich, 1980) on provider–patient interaction. It is likely that the orientation taken by the health-care provider will serve as systemic input and will influence the throughput process and outputs.

Finally, future health communication research could also benefit by a more specific application of a cybernetic systemic view. Because cybernetics emphasizes control, change, and feedback, such an application may help us work toward the outcome of improved health. The area of health communication is in a unique position within the field of communication, because it has as its goal measurable physiological outcomes. Unfortunately much of our research does not yet follow the system through to this natural outcome. That certainly is an important direction for further research.

REFERENCES

Aasterud, M. (1965). Explanation to the patient. In J. K. Skipper & R. C. Leonard (Eds.), *Social interaction and patient care.* Philadelphia: J. B. Lippincott.

Adler, K. (1977). Doctor–patient communication: A shift to problem-oriented research. *Human Communication Research, 3,* 179–190.

Aguilera, D. C. (1967). Relationship between physical contact and verbal interaction between nurses and patients. *Journal of Psychiatric Nursing, 5,* 5–12.

Albrecht, T. L. (1982). Coping with occupational stress: Relational and individual strategies of nurses in acute health care settings. In M. Burgoon (Ed.), *Communication yearbook 6* (pp. 832–849). New Brunswick, NJ: Transaction.

Albrecht, T. L., & Adelman, M. B. (1987). *Communicating social support.* Beverly Hills, CA: Sage.

Arntson, P., Droge, D., & Fassi, H. E. (1978). Pediatrician–patient communication: Final report. In B. D. Ruben (Ed.), *Communication yearbook 2* (pp. 505–522). New Brunswick, NJ: Transaction.

Aydelotte, M. K. (1960). *An investigation of the relation between nursing activity and patient welfare.* Ames, IA: State University of Iowa Press.

Barnard, D. (1985). Unsung questions of medical ethics. *Social Science and Medicine, 21,* 243–249.

Baziak, A. T., & Denton, R. K. (1960). The language of the hospital and its effects on the patient. *ETC; A Review of General Semantics, 17,* 261–268.

Ben-Sira, Z. (1980). Affective and instrumental components in the physician–patient relationship: An additional dimension of interaction theory. *Journal of Health and Social Behavior, 21,* 170–180.

Bird, B. (1955). *Talking with patients.* Philadelphia: Lippincott.

Brenders, D. A. (1986, July). *Perceived control and the interpersonal dimension of health care.* Paper presented at the Summer Conference on Health Education and Promotion in Primary care, Oxford, England.

Broadmore, J., Carr-Gregg, M., & Hutton, J. D. (1986). Vaginal examinations: Women's experiences and preferences. *New Zealand Medical Journal, 99,* 8–10.

Buchsbaum, D. G. (1986). Reassurance reconsidered. *Social Science and Medicine, 23,* 423–427.

Burgoon, M., Birk, T., Parrott, R., Coker, R., Pfau, M., & Burgoon, J. K. (1987, May). *Compliance-gaining strategy selection in physician–patient communication: I. Primary care physicians' perceptions.* Paper presented at the Annual Convention of the International Communication Association, Montreal.

Burgoon, M., Parrott, R., Coker, R., Birk, T., Pfau, M., & Burgoon, J. K. (1987, November). *Compliance-gaining strategy selection in physician–patient communication: II. Patients' perceptions.* Paper presented at the Annual Convention of the Speech Communication Association, Boston.

Carnerie, F. (1987). Crisis and informed consent: Analysis of a law-medicine malocclusion. *American Journal of Law and Medicine, 12,* 55–97.

Charney, E. (1972). Patient–doctor communication: Implications for the clinician. *Pediatrics Clinics of North America, 19,* 263–279.

Christman, L. P. (1966). Nurse–physician communication in the hospital. *International Nursing Review, 13,* 49–57.

Conrad, P. (1985). The meaning of medications: Another look at compliance. *Social Science and Medicine, 20,* 29–37.

Coulthard, M., & Ashby, M. (1975). Talking with the Doctor, 1. *Journal of Communication, 25,* 140–147.

Croft, J. J. (1980). Interviewing in physical therapy. *Physical Therapy, 60,* 1033–1036.

Crown, S. (1971). Failures of communication. *The Lancet, 7707,* 1021–1022.

Cunningham, M. A., & Wilcox, J. R. (1984). When an M.D. gives an R.N. a harmful order: Modifying a bind. In R. N. Bostrom (Ed.), *Communication yearbook 8* (pp. 764–778). Beverly Hills, CA: Sage.

Daly, M. B., & Hulka, B. S. (1975). Talking with the Doctor, 2. *Journal of Communication, 25,* 148–152.

Dance, F. E. X. (1970). The communication of health. *The Ohio Speech Journal, 8,* 28–30.

Dangott, L., Thornton, B. C., & Page, P. (1978). Communication and pain. *Journal of Communication, 28,* 30–35.

Davis, M. S. (1968). Variations in patients' compliance with doctor's advice: An empirical analysis of patterns of communication. *A.P.H.A., 58,* 274–288.

Davis, M. S. (1971). Variation in patients' compliance with doctors' order: Medical practice and doctor–patient interaction. *Psychiatric Medicine, 2,* 31.

Davison, R. (1985, August). *Ethical conflicts in medicine as a consequence of poor communication.* Paper presented at the Summer Conference on Health Communication, Evanston, IL.

Decastro, F. J. (1972). Doctor–patient communication: Exploring the effectiveness of care in a primary care clinic. *Clinical Pediatrics, 11,* 86–87.

Dervin, B., Harlock, S., Atwood, R., & Garzona, C. (1980). The human side of information: An exploration in a health communication context. In D. Nimmo (Ed.), *Communication yearbook 4* (pp. 591–608). New Brunswick, NJ: Transaction.

DiMatteo, M. R. (1979). A social-psychological analysis of physician–patient rapport: Toward a science of the art of medicine. *Journal of Social Issues, 35,* 12–33.

Dodge, J. S. (1965). Nurses' sense of adequacy and attitudes toward keeping patients informed. In J. K. Skipper & R. C. Leonard (Eds.), *Social interaction and patient care* (pp. 87–92). Philadelphia: J. B. Lippincott.

Dreyfuss, I. (1986, June 4). Anybody listening? *APA Newswire.*

Dumas, R. G., Anderson, B. J., & Leonard, R. C. (1965). The importance of the expressive function in preoperative preparation. In J. K. Skipper & R. C. Leonard (Eds.), *Social Interaction and patient care* (pp. 16–28). Philadelphia: J. B. Lippincott.

Egbert, L. D., Battit, G. E., Wilch, C. E., & Bartlett, M. K. (1964). Reduction of post operative pain by encouragement and instruction of patients. *New England Journal of Medicine, 270,* 825–827.

Elder, R. G. (1963). What is the patient saying, *Nursing Forum, 2,* 25–37.

Engel, G. L. (1973). *Interviewing the patient.* Philadelphia: W. B. Saunders.

Ferguson, K. J. (1987, June). *Patient participation and physician differences in patient–physician communication.* Paper presented at the Iowa Conference on Personal Relationships, Iowa City.

Francis, V., Korsch, B. M., & Morris, M. J. (1969). Gaps in doctor–patient communication: Patients' response to medical advice. *New England Journal of Medicine, 280,* 535–540.

Friedman, H. S. (1979). Nonverbal communication between patients and medical practitioners. *Journal of Social Issues, 35,* 82–99.

Friedman, H. S., & DiMatteo, M. R. (1979). Health care as an interpersonal process. *Journal of Social Issues, 35,* 1–11.

Fuller, D. S., & Quesada, G. M. (1973). Communication in medical therapeutics. *Journal of Communication, 23,* 361–370.

Gregg, D. (1965). Reassurance. In J. K. Skipper & R. C. Leonard (Eds.), *Social interaction and patient care* (pp. 127–136). Philadelphia: J. B. Lippincott.

Hawes, L. C. (1972a). Development and application of an interview coding system. *Central States Speech Journal, 23*, 92–99.

Hawes, L. C. (1972b). The effects of interviewer style on patterns of dyadic communication. *Speech Monographs, 39*, 114–123.

Hawes, L. C. (1973). A Markov analysis of interview communication. *Speech Monographs, 40*, 208–219.

Helfer, R. E., & Ealy, K. F. (1972). Observations of pediatric interviewing skills. *American Journal of Diseases of Children, 123*, 556–560.

Heszen-Klemens, I., & Lapinska, E. (1984). Doctor–patient interaction, patients' health behavior, and effects of treatment. *Social Science and Medicine, 19*, 9–18.

Hoffman, S. A. (1988, February). The doctor as dramatist. *Newsweek*, p. 10.

Hughes, J. (1980). Manipulation: A negative element in care. *Journal of Advanced Nursing, 5*, 21–29.

Jan, H. R. (1964). General semantic orientation in dentist–patient relations. *Journal of the American Dental Association, 68*, 424–429.

Kalisch, B. J. (1971). An experiment in the development of empathy in nursing students. *Nursing Research, 20*, 202–211.

Kaplan, A. (1964). *The conduct of inquiry: Methodology for the behavioral sciences*. New York: Chandler.

Kitson, A. L. (1987). A comparative analysis of lay-caring and professional (nursing) caring relationships. *International Journal of Nursing Studies, 24*, 155–165.

Kline, S. L., & Ceropski, J. M. (1985). Person-centered communication in medical practice. In G. M. Phillips & J. T. Wood (Eds.), *Emergent issues in human decision-making* (pp. 120–141). Carbonale: Southern Illinois University Press.

Korsch, B. M., Gozzi, E. K., & Francis, V. (1968). Gaps in doctor–patient communication: Doctor–patient interaction and patient satisfaction. *Pediatrics, 42*, 855–871.

Korsch, B. M., Freeman, B., & Negrete, V. F. (1971). Practical implications of doctor–patient interaction analyses for pediatric practice. *American Journal of Diseases of Children, 121*, 110–114.

Korsch, B. M., & Negrete, V. F. (1972). Doctor–patient communication. *Scientific America, 227*, 66–74.

Kreps, G. L. (1981). Nonverbal communication in dentistry. *The Dental Assistant, 50*, 18–20.

Kupst, M. J., Dresser, K., Schulman, J. L., & Paul, M. H. (1975). Evaluation of methods to improve communication in the physician–patient relationship. *American Journal of Orthopsychiatry, 45*, 420–429.

Lane, S. D. (1983). Compliance, satisfaction, and physician–patient communication. In R. N. Bostrom (Ed.), *Communication yearbook 7* (pp. 772–801). Beverly Hills, CA: Sage.

Levine, B. A., Moss, K. C., Ramsey, P. H., & Fleishman, R. A. (1978). Patient compliance with advice as a function of communicator expertise. *Journal of Social Psychology, 104*, 309–310.

Levy, D. R. (1985). White doctors and black patients: Influence of race on the doctor–patient relationship. *Pediatrics, 75*, 639–643.

Ley, P., & Spelman, M. S. (1967). *Communicating with the patient*. London: Trinity Press.

Liptak, G. S., Hulka, B. S., & Cassel, J. C. (1977). Effectiveness of physician–mother interactions during infancy. *Pediatrics, 60*, 186–192.

Lochman, J. E. (1983). Factors related to patients' satisfaction with their medical care. *Journal of Community Health, 9*, 91–109.

Logan, M. H., & Hunt, E. E., Jr. (1978). *Health and the human condition: Perspectives on medical anthropology*. North Scituate, MA: Duxbury press.

Long, K. A. (1985). Pitfalls to avoid and positive approaches in the nurse–adolescent relationship. *Perspectives in Psychiatric Care, 23*, 22–26.

Lucas, I. R. (1985, August). *The effects of initial interaction on uncertainty, rapport, and interpersonal attraction*. Paper presented at the Summer Conference on Health Communication, Evanston, IL.

Mace, D. R. (1971). Communication, interviewing, and the physician–patient relationship. In R. H. Coombs & C. E. Vincent (Eds.), *Psychosocial aspects of medical training* (pp. 380–408). Springfield, IL: Charles C. Thomas.

Malone, M., Berkowitz, N. H., & Klein, M. W. (1962). Interpersonal conflict in the outpatient department. *American Journal of Nursing, 62*, 108–112.

Marks, J. N., Goldberg, D. P., & Hillier, V. F. (1979). Determinants of the ability of general practitioners to detect psychiatric illness. *Psychological Medicine, 9*, 337–353.

Matthews, D. A., Sledge, W. H., & Lieberman, P. B. (1987). Evaluation of intern performance by medical inpatients. *American Journal of Medicine, 83*, 938–944.

May, M. L. (1985, August). *Patients and doctors in conflict: The nature of patients' complaints and what they do about them*. Paper presented at the Summer Conference on Health Communication, Evanston, IL.

Mayo, N. E. (1978). Patient compliance: Practical implications for physical therapists. *Physical Therapy, 58*, 1083–1090.

Meize-Grochowski, R. (1984). An analysis of the concept of trust. *Journal of Advanced Nursing, 9*, 563–572.

Meyers, M. E. (1965). The effect of types of communication on patients' reactions to stress. In J. K. Skipper & R. C. Leonard (Eds.), *Social interaction and patient care*. Philadelphia: J. B. Lippincott.

Miller, W. D. (1975). Drug usage: Compliance of patients with instructions on medicine. *Journal of American Osteopath Association, 75*, 401–404.

Molleman, E., Krabbendam, P. J., Annyas, A. A., Koops, H. S., Sleijfer, D. T., & Vermey, A. (1984). The significance of the doctor–patient relationship in coping with cancer. *Social Science and Medicine, 18*, 475–480.

Moore, L. G., Van Arsdale, P. W., Glittenberg, J. E., & Aldrich, R. A. (1980). *The biocultural basis of health: The expanding views of medical anthropology*. St. Louis: C. V. Mosby.

Morse, B. W., & Piland, R. N. (1981). An assessment of communication competencies needed by intermediate-level health care providers: A study of nurse–patient, nurse–doctor, and nurse–nurse communication relationships. *Journal of Advances in Consumer Research, 9*, 30–41.

Neal, J. (1962). *Better communications for better health*. New York: Columbia University Press.

New, P. K., Nite, G., & Callahan, J. M. (1959). *Nursing service and patient care: A staffing experiment*. Kansas City, MO: Community Studies.

Northouse, P. G. (1979). Interpersonal trust and empathy in nurse–nurse relationships. *Nursing Research, 28*, 365–368.

Nutting, P. A. (1986). Health promotion in primary medical care: Problems and potential. *Preventive Medicine, 15*, 537–548.

O'Hair, D. (1989). Dimensions of relational communication during physician and patient interactions. *Health Communication, 1*, 97–115.

Ort, R. S., Ford, A. B., & Liske, R. E. (1964). The doctor–patient relationship as described by physicians and medical students. *Journal of Health and Human Behavior, 5*, 25–33.

Parsons, T. (1951). *The social system*. New York: The Free Press.

Plainfield, S. (1969). Communication distortion: The language of patient practitioners of dentistry. *Journal of Prosthetic Dentistry, 22,* 11–19.

Powers, J. S. (1985). Patient–physician communication and interaction: A unifying approach to the difficult patient, *Southern Medical Journal, 78,* 445–447.

Pruyn, J. F. A., Ruckman, R. M., van Brunschot, C. J. M., & van de Borne, H. W. (1985). Cancer patients' personality characteristics, physician–patient communication and adoption of the Moerman diet. *Social Science and Medicine, 20,* 841–847.

Raimbault, G., Cachin, O., Limal, C., Eliacheff, C., & Rappaport, R. (1975). Aspects of communication between patients and doctors: An analysis of the discourse in medical interviews. *Pediatrics, 55,* 401–405.

Ray, E. B., & Bostrom, R. N. (1987). *The relationship of physician gender, patient gender, and seriousness of illness on patient recall.* Paper presented at the Annual Convention of the Speech Communication Association, Boston, MA.

Reader, G., Pratt, L., & Mudd, M. (1957). What patients expect from their doctors. *Modern Hospital, 89,* 88–94.

Redland, A. R. (1983, May). *An investigation of nurses' interaction styles with physicians and suggested patient care interventions.* Paper presented at the Annual Convention of the International Communication Association, Dallas.

Rochelle, P. (1966). How to answer questions. *Physical Therapy, 46,* 428.

Rodin, J., & Janis, I. L. (1979). The social power of health-care practitioners as agents of change. *Journal of Social Issues, 35,* 60–81.

Roter, D. L. (1984). Patient question asking in physician–patient interaction. *Health Psychology, 3,* 395–409.

Rubin, F. L., Judd, M. M., & Conine, T. A. (1977). Empathy: Can it be learned and retained? *Physical therapy, 57,* 644–647.

Rubin, R. L. (1986). Assisting adolescents toward mental health. *Nursing Clinics of North America, 21,* 439–450.

Samora, J., Saunders, L., & Larson, R. F. (1961). Medical vocabulary knowledge among hospital patients. *Journal of Health and Human Behavior, 2,* 83–92.

Sanger, J. O. (1964). The rudiments of public speaking. *Physical Therapy, 44,* 290–293.

Schwartz, L. R., & Overton, D. T. (1987). Emergency department complaints: A one-year analysis. *Annuals of Emergency Medicine, 16,* 847–860.

Shulman, B. H., Peven, D., & Byrne, A. (1973). Graffiti therapy. *Hospital and Community Psychiatry, 24,* 339–340.

Simoni, J. J., & Ball, R. A. (1975). Can we learn from medicine hucksters? *Journal of Communication, 25,* 174–181.

Skipper, J. K. (1965a). Communication and the hospitalized patients. In J. K. Skipper & R. C. Leonard (Eds.), *Social interaction and patient care* (pp. 61–81). Philadelphia: J. B. Lippincott.

Skipper, J. K. (1965b). The role of the hospital nurse: Is it instrumental or expressive? In J. K. Skipper & R. C. Leonard (Eds.), *Social interaction and patient care* (pp. 40–50). Philadelphia: J. B. Lippincott.

Spaan, R. C. (1964). A tooth is a tooth . . . Aristotle: A tooth is not a tooth . . . Korzybski. *Journal of the Oklahoma Dental Association, 68,* 424–429.

Special Communication. Professional crisis—Can physical therapists afford not to communicate? (1977). *Physical Therapy, 57,* 409–410.

Stone, G. C. (1979). Patient compliance and the role of the expert. *Journal of Social Issues, 35,* 34–59.

Street, R. L., & Wiemann, J. M. (1987). Patient satisfaction with physicians' interpersonal involvement, expressiveness, and dominance. In M. L. McLaughlin (Ed.), *Communication yearbook 10* (pp. 591–612). Beverly Hills, CA: Sage.

Swiderski, R. M. (1976). The idiom of diagnosis. *Communication Quarterly, 24,* 3–11.

Tarasuk, M. B., Rhymes, J. P., & Leonard, R. C. (1965). An experimental test of the importance of communication skills for effective nursing. In J. K. Skipper & R. C. Leonard (Eds.), *Social interaction and patient care* (pp. 110–120). Philadelphia: J. B. Lippincott.

Thompson, T. L. (1984). The invisible helping hand: The role of communication in the health and social service professions. *Communication Quarterly, 32,* 148–163.

Thompson, T. L. (1986). *Communication for health professionals: A relational perspective.* New York: Harper & Row.

Toombs, S. K. (1987). The meaning of illness: A phenomenological approach to the patient–physician relationship. *Journal of Medicine and Philosophy, 12,* 219–240.

Trandel-Korenchuk, D. M. (1987). The effect of social and care environments on the disclosure practices of nurse midwives relative to methods of pain management in childbirth. *Journal of Obstetric, Gynecologic & Neonatal Nursing, 16,* 258–265.

Tryon, P. A., & Leonard, R. C. (1965). Giving the patient an active role. In J. K. Skipper & R. C. Leonard (Eds.), *Social interaction and patient care* (pp. 120–127). Philadelphia: J. B. Lippincott.

Villard, K. L., & Whipple, L. N. (1974). *Beginnings in relational communication.* New York: Wiley.

Vowles, K. O. (1970). *Development of a communication course for undergraduate dental students.* Unpublished master's thesis, San Francisco State College, San Francisco, CA.

Wain, H. A. (1970). *A history of preventive medicine.* Springfield, IL: Charles C. Thomas.

Walker, H. L. (1973). Communication and the American health care problem. *Journal of Communication, 23,* 349–360.

Willmington, R. A., & Willmington, S. C. (1988). *What research says to the nurse communicator.* Unpublished manuscript, Marian College of Fond du Lac, Fond du Lac, WI.

Worobey, J. L., & Cummings, H. W. (1984). Communication effectiveness of nurses in four relational settings. *Journal of Applied Communication Research, 12,* 128–141.

Young, W. O., & Smith, L. (1972). The nature and organization of dental practice. In H. Freeman (Ed.), *Handbook of Medical Sociology* (2nd ed., pp. 231–249). Englewood Cliffs, NJ: Prentice-Hall.

4

The Health Caregiver–
Patient Relationship:
Pathology, Etiology,
Treatment

Brent D. Ruben
Rutgers University

The relationship between human communication and health care is a very fundamental one. Communication is the process through which symptoms are described and interpreted, and the means through which treatment is provided and compliance encouraged. It is the mechanism through which scientific advances are shared within the research and professional community, the vehicle through which medical personnel are trained and patients educated, and the link through which caregivers from different specialties interact with one another on a daily basis. Moreover, the process of communication is central to the way individuals and societies conceptualize and cope with illness.

At the heart of the linkage between communication and health care, and the focus of this chapter, is the nature of the relationship between caregivers and patients. This relationship has become an increasing focus of attention in recent years in major works in both the popular and academic press (e.g., Shorter, 1985; Siegel, 1986; Sneider, 1986; Tuckett, Boulton, Olson, & Williams, 1985; West, 1984). The interest in this relationship is reflective of a number of factors, not the least of which is a growing recognition of the critical functions of caregiver–patient communication in various facets of health care (Cline, 1983; Cline & Cardosi, 1983; Ernstene, 1957; Kleinman, 1980; Korsch & Gozzi, 1968; Korsch & Negrete, 1972; Kreps & Thornton, 1984; Lane, 1983; Mechanic, 1982; Northouse & Northouse, 1985; Ruben & Bowman, 1986; Thompson, 1984; Waitzkin, 1984; Wertz, Sorenson, & Heeren, 1988; Woolley, Kane, Hughes, & Wright, 1978).

Unfortunately the caregiver–patient relationship is as problematic as it is important, embodying all the complexity and challenge—and even greater stress—than is present in other professional–lay relationships. As with the teacher and student, the attorney and client, or the librarian and the information seeker, the relationship between the caregiver and the patient is characteristically asymmetrical in that expertise and power are unevenly distributed. And although both parties to such relationships can be said to have a common purpose—to be independent components of a common system[1]–they seldom share common perspectives.

For their part, physicians, nurses, and allied health-care staff participate in the relationship as knowledgeable professionals, "at home" in the environment in which the interactions are occurring, seeing patients on a schedule that they set. They are familiar with terminology and protocols, able to routinely take medical histories and perform necessary physical exams and diagnostic procedures, and generally have substantial experience with the range of medical problems and circumstances that present themselves.

Patients, on the other hand, come to the relationship looking for help in some form. They do so in an environment that is unfamiliar, one that they often perceive as intimidating. Patients must schedule the encounter at the convenience of the caregivers, and often have to wait to be seen. Frequently they enter the interaction anxious about their health, and lacking medical knowledge or relevant professional expertise. For the patient, even "routine" history-taking, physical exams, and tests are discomforting. This is a consequence of the necessity for levels of verbal disclosure and physical contact normally reserved for intimate relationships. And, depending on the outcome of these encounters, patients may be faced with the need to comply with recommendations for behavioral change, undergo additional testing, or accept continuing uncertainty about their health status.

ASSESSING SYSTEM FUNCTIONING:
DEFINING QUALITY OF CARE

One of the most significant manifestations of the lack of integration between components of caregiver–patient systems can be seen in the respective criteria used in assessing the quality of system functioning.

Given a shared goal of improving health care, one might assume

---

[1]Detailed discussions of the communication systems concepts underlying the framework presented in this chapter are provided in Allport, 1955; Blumer, 1966; Bochner & Kelly, 1974; Miller, 1965; Ruben, 1972, 1978, 1983a, 1983b; Ruben & Kealey, 1979; Ruben & Kim, 1975; Ruesch & Bateson, 1951; Selye, 1956; Thayer, 1968; and elsewhere in this volume.

that caregivers and patients would evaluate the functioning of health-care systems in essentially the same way, using the same or a similar framework. This seems not to be the case. Evidence suggests that for the most part medical personnel base their assessments of quality of care on clinical and technical criteria: Have correct diagnostic procedures been followed? Were appropriate treatment protocols adhered to? Was testing conducted in a technically correct manner? (Droste, 1988; Siegel, 1986; Steiber, 1988)

As Siegel (1986) explained:

> I'd been trained to think my whole job was doing things to people in a mechanical way to make them better, to save their lives. This is how a doctor's success is defined. (p. 11)
>
> I'd been dealing in cases, charts, diseases, remedies, staff, and progno ses, . . . I'd thought of my patients . . . as machines I had to repair. (p. 14)

Thus, it is generally the case that caregivers make their assessments of quality of care based on clinical and technical criteria, clinical and technical skills or competencies of providers, and the manner in which patients are treated *medically*. Patients, family members, and friends lack the expertise to make judgments in this same manner. Their assessments of quality are, understandably, less technical and clinical in nature, emphasizing communication-oriented criteria, caregiver's communication competence, and the manner in which they are treated *personally* (Korsch & Negrete, 1972; Ruben & Bowman, 1986; Ruben & Ruben, 1988; Steiber, 1988).

Ruben and Bowman (Ruben, 1986); and Ruben and Ruben (1988) have addressed the question of patient evaluative criteria directly through surveys to random samples of 1,000 former patients from each of several major community hospitals 6 months after discharge. The most relevant findings for illustrating the point in question are results from the content analysis of the open-ended responses to a portion of the survey in which patients were asked to relate their most memorable experience at the hospital. Respondents were requested to: "Think back on your stay at the hospital. Please describe, in a sentence of two, your most memorable positive or negative experience. (This can be any experience related to the hospital, its staff, or its services.)" Table 4.1 provides a listing of coding categories that were developed and a summary of the frequency of responses for each category for two hospitals.

While many patients related incidents associated with the quality of clinical and technical care (particularly in instances of a negative incident), more memorable incidents mentioned involved staff communication skills and personal treatment. And, as is apparent from

TABLE 4.1
Factors Associated with Patients' Most Remembered Experiences
During Hospitalization*

Factor	Number of Experiences Reported	Percentage of All Experiences
Personal treatment/Interpersonal communication skill	216	44.2
Quality of clinical care	171	35.0
Facility/environment	29	6.0
Policies and procedures	25	5.1
Information provided	20	4.1
Food	9	1.8
Other	19	3.9
TOTAL	489	100.1

*Based on content analysis and classification of open-ended responses

Table 4.1, other "nonclinical" factors such as facilities, policies, and procedures, and information also play an important role in patient evaluations.

Examples of the responses are provided in Tables 4.2, 4.3, 4.4, 4.5, and 4.6, organized according to the five emergent coding categories: (a) personal treatment/interpersonal communication; (b) quality of clinical care; (c) facilities; (d) policies and procedures; and (e) adequacy of information provided.

The importance of the personal treatment to patient assessments of quality of care was also highlighted in a recent Gallup/Hospitals Poll. The study reported that for patients "concern from staff" was the factor most highly correlated with "quality" ($r=.60$). Items more closely related to clinical and technical issues, such as "physician care" and "nursing care," also correlated with "quality" assessments but at lower levels ($r=.44$ and $r=.55$, Steiber, 1988).

Apparent differences in the criteria used by caregivers and patients to assess the quality of system functioning provide additional evidence of the lack of shared evaluative criteria, and at the same time underscore the need for a more systemic framework in terms of which to conceive of the caregiver–patient relationship.

THE INTERCULTURAL NATURE OF THE CAREGIVER–PATIENT RELATIONSHIP

These and other discontinuities in the caregiver–patient relationship present difficulties and challenges that manifest themselves in virtually every facet of caregiver–patient interaction. We have come increasingly to recognize that this lack of integration is not the result of a

TABLE 4.2
Patients' Most Memorable Experiences:
Representative Responses Related to
Personal Treatment/Interpersonal Communication Skill

Positive Statements:

"I found everyone to be very cheerful and always plesant to be with, which really helps when you're staying in a strange place."

"Without exception, the nurses went out of their way to be friendly."

"Warmth and concern were shown by nurses and staff to me. I felt as though I was a person, not just a name on the chart or a clinical case to be analyzed."

"Without exception, everyone on the floor took care of my father as if he were their father."

"I have the highest regard for nurses and staff in the maternity ward. They left me with a positive attitude toward birth."

Negative Statements:

"The 3 p.m. to 11 p.m. nurse on Maternity is a bitch! No compassion."

"Staff discusses patients openly to other staff, affording anyone in a nearby room an ear-full."

"Many technicians, in my opinion, lacked compasion and concern. They also had no respect for my dignity or modesty. A friendly smile would have helped. They did what they were trained to do and that's all."

"Need more attentive and listening doctors and nurses."

"The weekend floor nurses stink—they do not respond, are rude and do not give a damn about your feelings."

TABLE 4.3
Patients' Most Memorable Experiences:
Representative Responses Related to
Clinical/Technical Quality of Care

Positive Statements:

"Through six major surgical procedures I have always felt that I had the best possible medical care at all times."

"Staff and services are very organized . . . I was very well taken care of . . . "

Negative Statements:

"The floor physician and nurses on night shift are very incompetent—they were unable to insert an I.V. in patients' arms correctly."

"The RN almost gave my infection medicine to my roomate who was very allergic to it."

"I.V. was moved back and forth to either arm at least five times."

"The doctor in the E.R. room was rushed and inconsiderate. To this day (3 years later), I have chronic pain from an injury. I think I was diagnosed wrong."

TABLE 4.4
Patients' Most Memorable Experiences:
Representative Responses Related to Facilities/Environment

Positive Statements:

"Very clean, well run, efficient institution."
"The birthing room facilities were peaceful and beautiful."
"I think _____ is the best hospital around. It is clean and nurses are kind and considerate."

Negative Statements:

"The rooms by the nursing stations should be lounges. Definitely too noisy."
"I'm very dissatisfied with your parking. . . ."
"Bathrooms could be kept cleaner."

TABLE 4.5
Patients' Most Memorable Experiences: Related to
Policies and Procedures

Positive Statements:

"Attention given to siblings of newborns is a nice touch."

Negative Statements:

"Dinner trays are brought too early."
"When being discharged, the procedures are too involved."
"There should be some afternoon visitation for those people who work evening hours."

TABLE 4.6
Patients' Most Memorable Experiences:
Representative Responses Related to Information Provided

Positive Statements:

"The anesthetist went out of his way before surgery to allay my fears."
"The night before my operation the doctor explained the operation to me. This relaxed me."
"I liked the way that all the nurses and doctors took the time to explain the heart catherization test to me."

Negative Statements:

"First day—no information given at all. Very frustrating."
"The emergency room should keep you informed as to why you are lying there for so long."
"One attending (full-time staff) doctor always swept in and out leaving me no chance to ask questions. I felt as though I did not exist."

simple communication problem—the kind that can be solved with minor improvements to information systems, attention to clearer speaking, more repetition of instructions by caregivers, or another educational pamphlet for patients (Allaire & McNeil, 1983; American Board of Internal Medicine, 1979; Bertakis, 1977; Korsch & Gozzi, 1968; Korsch & Negrete, 1972; Physicians for the Twenty-First Century, 1984; Ruben & Ruben, 1988; Shorter, 1985). These are, rather, far more fundamental communication problems, more appropriately termed *communication pathologies,* that occur in interactions between representatives of what are essentially very different worlds—worlds that share a common purpose, but seldom a common perspective.

As with other professional–lay relationships (where purposes may be common, but perspectives, system criteria, and evaluative frameworks, are not) what we have in the case of the caregiver–patient relationship is essentially an intercultural relationship (Brislin, 1981; Ellingsworth, 1977; Gudykunst & Kim, 1984; Kim, 1988; Ruben, 1976, 1983b, 1985b).

The term *intercultural* refers to a circumstance in which interpersonal communication requires the bridging of two distinct cultures, each with its own characteristic symbols, meanings, conventions, rule structures, habits, values, communication patterns, social realities, and "significant stories," that are shared in common by members of a particular social system or subsystem (Ruben, 1983, 1988b). Each social system or subsystem evolves its own system culture that serves to distinguish it in subtle and sometimes not so subtle ways from other social systems (Ruben, 1983). As individuals learn, adapt to, and/or adapt the cultures of these social systems, their behavior at once confirms, validates, and transmits that culture to others in the social system (Ruben, 1983b). The result is that over time individuals develop the necessary "tools of the trade" to participate in the cultures and subcultures of the subsystems—relationships, groups, organizations, and societies.

Through this fundamental, pervasive yet subtle communication process, physicians become physicians, hospital volunteers become volunteers, nurses become nurses, health-care administrators become administrators, and patients become patients. To the extent that physicians, nurses, volunteers, and administrators become enculturated into their own subsystem cultures, the interaction between them and patients is essentially intercultural communication.

From this perspective, we have a view of a health-care worker who is professionally educated, speaking a familiar language, and using familiar tools. The caregiver encounters patients in a familiar environment that he or she understands and to which he or she has adapted.

It is a place of work, a place where his or her professional and technical training can be practiced, and a context one shares with peers with shared outlooks.

Most patients and visitors, lacking a similar education, language capability, and familiarity with the tools, experience this same environment as unfamiliar, alien, and frightening. What is routine to a hospital staff is generally a crisis for a patient. And in the case of hospitalization, the usual problems of loss of control and anxiety associated with adjusting to a strange cultural situation or circumstance are substantially magnified (Furnham & Bichner, 1986; Gudykunst & Kim, 1984; Hall, 1959; Kim, 1988; Ruben 1983b). In this framework, it seems quite clear that the difficulties of negotiating common understandings and commitments to action across these cultural boundaries are substantial.

An awareness that subsystems have their own unique cultures is a useful notion with major implications for diagnosing pathology in interpersonal health-care systems. Indeed, one of the most parsimonious explanations for the interpersonal communication difficulties that occur in caregiver–patient encounters, is simply that communication between caregiver and patient is, above all else, an instance of intercultural (more correctly intersubcultural) communication—communication between representatives of two quite different subsystems, living in what are essentially two very different realities, who bring different backgrounds, expectations, understandings, knowledge, sensitivities (and insensitivities), communication behaviors, and interpretative conventions to the interaction.

OVERCOMING SYSTEM–CULTURE BARRIERS

Competitive Influences

Few fields have undergone the rapid change that has characterized the health-care industry in recent years. The combined impact of the increased competition within the health-care industry, new medical technology and procedures, increased public scrutiny, better informed patients, heightened expectations for service and quality, new diseases, and the economics of health care has been dramatic on health-care workers at all levels.

Collectively, demands on workers to be more productive, cost-conscious, technologically competent, and marketing oriented are often mentioned as having exacerbated barriers to improvements in caregiver–patient relationships. Although these developments are additional sources of stress for health-care workers, ironically, the same changes in the marketplace have also provided an impetus for the adoption of a more integrated view of health-care systems. Indeed, it has been noted that one of the potentially very positive byproducts of the competition and complexity that increasingly characterizes the health-care environment is a growing emphasis on patient satisfaction (Ruben & Bowman, 1986).

From a systems perspective, this outcome is not surprising. To the extent that health-care systems strive to adapt in a competitive environment where consumers have a broadened range of choice, survival increasingly depends on consumer satisfaction and on repeat and referral business. As the number of alternative health-care facilities and services grow, administrators recognize that patient impressions of the care they receive play an increasingly central role in their selection of providers and provider institutions. Obviously, a person who has a positive experience with a particular physician, HMO, or clinic will be likely to choose the same provider in the future when need dictates— and will suggest that others in his or her social networks do so as well. Conversely, the dissatisfied individual would be far more likely to explore alternatives. And given that negativism and dissatisfaction are diffused far more widely than satisfaction—the "multiplier" or "ripple" effect—the impact of dissatisfied patients is recognized as being substantial from a variety of points of view (Leebov, 1988; Lewis, 1983; Ruben, 1985a). Thus, in today's health-care environment, patient satisfaction is tied to the economic bottomline of hospitals and other health-care organizations more directly than at any previous time, an awareness that is leading health-care administrators to press for greater attention by caregivers to the concerns and evaluative criteria used by patients and visitors (Leebov, 1988; Ruben, 1985a; Ruben & Bowman, 1986).

Intervention Strategies: Enhancing Communication Competencies Through Education and Training

In addition to the natural influence of competitive pressures toward greater integration of the caregiver–patient perspectives, purposeful intervention strategies are also available as a means of addressing the complexities and challenges inherent in caregiver–patient relationships.

Because many of the barriers to improved health-care relationships are characteristic of intercultural relationships in general, essentially the goal of intervention strategies is to enhance the competencies of representatives from one cultural system to better understand and relate effectively with representatives of the other. We can identify three essential classes, or clusters, of communication competencies[2] that have potential to contribute to this goal.

They are:

- *Information-Transfer Competencies.* These competencies refer to verbal and nonverbal coding and decoding abilities associated with the transmission and reception of information with minimum loss and distortion.
- *Relationship Development and Maintenance Competencies.* This second class refers to the development of rapport, establishment of credibility and trust, demonstration of empathy and respect, and interaction management.
- *Compliance-Gaining Competencies.* These competencies refer to the abilities that are necessary to persuasion and to securing an appropriate level of compliance and/or cooperation.

Taking this framework as a point of departure, there are two types of intervention strategies available—strategies designed to foster an improved communicative relationship through enhanced patient communication competencies, and those designed to help improve caregiver communication competencies.

Patient Communication Competence and Patient Education

It is generally agreed that the public today is better educated with respect to health care than at any previous time. However, even with increased information sources, new information technologies, and the increasing emphasis being placed on health-care–consumer education, advances in medical science and technology on the "provider side" seem likely to perpetuate the knowledge gap between medical professionals and patients.

There remain many examples of areas where a lack of knowledge and inappropriate attitudes toward health and disease are still major impediments to improved health care (Kreps, Ruben, Baker, & Rosenthal, 1987; Ruben, 1986b). And, an unwillingness, inability, or reluc-

---

[2]It is beyond the scope of this chapter to provide a detailed examination of the concept of communication competence. Such discussions are provided in Bochner & Kelly, 1974; Bostrom, 1984; Kelly, 1979; Ruben, 1976, 1988b; Ruben & Kealey, 1979; Spitzberg & Cupach, 1984; Wiemann & Backlund, 1980.

tance to utilize health information can be a problem not only for patients, but also for health-care providers (Kreps, Hubbard, & DeVita, 1988; Ruben, 1986).

Notwithstanding this caveat, it seems clear that this higher level of awareness and knowledge of health and health-related topics has obvious potential to contribute to increasingly productive and satisfying caregiver–patient relationships (Kreps, this volume). Today, as in the earliest days of medical care, the heart of health care is the provider–patient relationship. It is at this interface that the adverse consequences of a cultural knowledge gap are most apparent, and it is in this connection that health education holds great promise. When successful, health education efforts can be particularly valuable for enhancing patient information-transfer competence as a result of broadening patients' understanding and familiarity with the terminology, perspective, and concepts of the caregiver culture (Sneider, 1986). This knowledge may lead to improved patient comprehension and more informed questioning. In some instances, increased knowledge may also be of assistance to patients indirectly in their efforts to establish rapport and credibility with caregivers.

Generally speaking, increased information alone, however, is less likely to be of direct value as it relates to relationship building and maintenance and compliance gaining. In some circumstances, increased levels of patient information may actually inhibit rather than enhance relationship development and maintenance endeavors of patients, if utilized in a manner that is perceived as inappropriately challenging or threatening by caregivers who themselves may lack relationship-building and maintenance competence. Moreover, increased knowledge is likely to be of little consequence in patients' attempts to encourage caregiver accommodation of their information needs, concerns, scheduling constraints, and the like.

A means of addressing relationship-building and maintenance and compliance competencies for patients more directly is suggested by implication in the research protocol used by Greenfield and Kaplan (Greenfield, Kaplan, & Ware, 1985, 1986; Kaplan, Ware, & Greenfield, 1986). In essence, the Greenfield and Kaplan approach consists of meeting with patients prior to their appointments with their physician in a session designed to help them review their medical record, coach them in formulating relevant questions, and assist them in rehearsing techniques for negotiating medical decisions with their physicians.

By implication, results from this research are most interesting from the perspective of patient competency. They indicate that as a result of the experimental manipulation, patients reported fewer limitations in their physical and role-related activities, were more effective in obtaining information, developed an increased preference for active involvement in medical decision making, and were as satisfied with their interaction with physicians as patients who did not undergo this preparation (Greenfield et al., 1985). Other studies have indicated that the effects of this intervention technique extend beyond improvements in self-reported assessments of the quality of functioning and observations of differences in communication patterns in interactions with physicians, and in fact have led to physiological changes (e.g., improved blood sugar control among diabetics; Greenfield et al., 1986).

Findings from these studies also lend credence to the earlier observation that increased levels of information alone are unlikely to contribute to relationship development and compliance gaining. Patients in the control group in the Greenfield and Kaplan studies, where the outcomes just mentioned did not occur, followed what can be characterized as a more traditional information-transmission model of patient education (Ruben, 1988a). These patients met with a medical assistant who reviewed information on their particular disease, including information about its cause, complications, and treatment. Absent from the control group were discussions of their own medical history, consideration of behavior-change strategies, and opportunities to rehearse questions and question asking. While awaiting additional testing and development, it appears that educational strategies utilizing active involvement and simulated interaction, combined with the presentation of patient-specific information, have excellent potential as tools for enhancing patient communication competencies, and the quality and value of their interactions with caregivers.

Caregiver Communication Competence
and Patient/Guest Relations Training

Communication competency training for caregivers is a conceptually similar strategy. The caregiver role, although traditionally associated primarily with the physician, and sometimes the nurse, refers increasingly today to an ever-broadening list of trained specialists within health-care institutions who interface with patients. This terminological change is motivated by both a changing concept and pragmatics of the marketplace. It is becoming clear that the communication competencies (or lack of them) of every health-care staff member who has contact with the patient or family member—and even some who do not have direct contact—may have a bearing on patient health care and satisfaction. Research findings suggest that lack of interpersonal skill by admitting staff, business office personnel, or maintenance staff can have as great an impact on patients' lasting impressions as the treatment provided by professional health-care staff (Ruben & Bowman, 1986; see Table 4.7).

Depending on the particular caregiver role involved, the relative importance of specific communication competencies varies. It has long been recognized that information-transmission competencies of clinical staff play a vital role in interactions with patients related to prevention, diagnosis, and treatment (Bertakis, 1977; Korsch & Gozzi, 1968; Korsch & Negrete, 1972; Stewart & Cash, 1985; Waitzkin, 1984, 1986; Wertz et al., 1988). Perhaps less obvious is that effective information transfer is not unimportant in interactions between other health-care personnel who have contact with patients (e.g., food service workers, business office staff, volunteers, or housekeeping staff). The informational content of some of these contacts may have direct consequence for health care in a clinical sense. Even where this is not the case, as noted previously, the quality of these interactions often has an impact on the patients' level of anxiety and sense of control, in their assessment of the quality of care, and in the impression that is formed of the provider institution (Ruben & Bowman, 1986).

The recognition that the quality of provider-patient relationships is exceedingly important to health care from a number of perspectives, points directly to the significance of relationship development and maintenance competencies (Cline, 1983; Cline & Cardosi, 1983; Ernstene, 1957; Fine & Therrien, 1977; Kaplan et al., 1986; Physicians for the Twenty-First Century, 1984; Shorter, 1985; Siegel, 1986; Thompson, 1984; Woolley et al., 1978). Aspects of relationship building such as the development of rapport, display of empathy, establishment of credibility and trust, beyond being of value in their own right, also often facilitate information transfer and compliance gaining (Ernstene,

TABLE 4.7
Caregiver Role and Valence Associated with Most Remembered
Experiences During Hospitalization*

	Positive References	Negative References	Total	Percent
Physicians	18	20	38	10.0
Nurses	129	41	170	44.7
Other staff	30	16	46	12.1
No role mentioned			126	33.2
TOTAL	177	187	380	100.0

*Based on content analysis and classification of open-ended responses from returns on 1,000 surveys to former patients at one hospital

1957; Fine & Therrien, 1977; Kaplan et al., 1986; Korsch & Gozzi, 1968; Korsch & Negrete, 1972; Lane, 1983; Siegel, 1986; Tuckett et al., 1985; Waitzkin, 1984, 1986).

Caregiver communication competence has been a topic of increasing concern, and a number of efforts have been undertaken to address this need. In the case of physicians one approach has been to introduce and/or extend the emphasis placed on communication in the formal education and certification programs (American Board of Internal Medicine, 1979; Physicians for the Twenty-First Century, 1984).

The introduction of what are called *Patient Relations Programs* (or Guest Relations or *Customer Relations Programs*) is another intervention strategy developed in part to address these needs for a broad range of caregivers. (Allaire & McNeil, 1983; Bowman & Ruben, 1986; Leebov, 1988; Ruben, 1985a; Ruben & Bowman, 1986)

Patient relations programs may be informational, experiential, or a combination thereof. Training may be designed for clinical and technical health-care staff, "front-line" support personnel, and/or service staff. Administrators may also participate (Allaire & McNeil, 1983; Bowman & Ruben, 1986; Leebov, 1988; Ruben, 1985a; Ruben & Bowman, 1986). The training goals, approach, format, and intended audiences vary from program to program. As described, such programs build on the goals of educational and professional development programs, while simultaneously addressing goals of organizational development, quality assurance, and marketing.

The goals of one patient relations program designed to emphasize communication competencies include: (a) Heightening staff sensitivity to the nature of the patient experience, including fear, confusion, loss of control, and lack of knowledge of procedures and terminology; (b) increasing staff understanding of the communication skills necessary to respond meaningfully to fundamental patient and family needs, including listening, empathy, nonverbal communication, coping with anxiety and hostility; (c) improving staff skills for developing and maintaining effective relationships with patients, family members, and co-workers, including creating rapport, demonstrating interpersonal sensitivity, establishing credibility, and building trust; and (d) enhancing understanding and cooperation across departments, specialties, and occupational groups, including heightening staff understanding of the health-care industry, involving staff at all levels, encouraging a sharing of perspectives, and fostering a sense of teamwork (Ruben, 1985a).

The effectiveness of training interventions such as patient or guest relations programs is, at best, difficult to assess. Moreover, it is well recognized that success in achieving program goals requires managerial support, a conducive culture, systematic follow-up, and regular reinforcement for the training program itself (Allaire & McNeil, 1983; Bowman & Ruben, 1986; Leebov, 1988). Available evaluation techniques include pre- and posttest surveys of former patients, pre- and posttest assessments of caregiver communication competencies, self-report by participants, and/or formalized assessments by supervisors (Bowman & Ruben, 1986; Ruben & Bowman, 1986; Ruben & Ruben, 1988).

CONCLUSION

Communication systems theory points to the importance of operating from what may be termed an integrated perspective on the health care system, one which recognizes the co-defining and intercultural nature of caregiver–patient relationships.

It has been suggested that in a great many instances the caregiver and patient subsystems—and resultant subcultures—utilize quite different criteria in assessing the quality of the system's performance. Clinical and technical criteria are emphasized in assessments within the caregiver subsystem. For patients and family members lacking the medical expertise on which to base assessments of the care provided, caregiver communication competencies often become the focus of evaluation.

Although the caregiver–patient relationship is an extremely complex and problematic one, intervention strategies emphasizing communication competency training for either or both role groups have potential to alleviate some of the inherent difficulties. Neither patient-based nor caregiver-based interventions should be viewed as a panacea; nonetheless, each represents a systematic approach to addressing what is certainly one of the most critical challenges facing health care today.

ACKNOWLEDGMENTS

The author gratefully acknowledges the suggestions of Gary Radford and Nurit Guttman during the preparation of this manuscript.

REFERENCES

Allaire, B., & McNeil, R. (1983). *Teaching patient relations in hospitals: The how's and why's*. Chicago: American Hospital Association.
Allport, G. W. (1955). *Becoming*. New Haven, CT: Yale University Press.
American Board of Internal Medicine. (1979). Clinical competence in internal medicine. *Annals of Internal Medicine, 90*(3), 402–411.

Bertakis, K. D. (1977). The communication of information from physician to patient: A method of increasing patient retention and satisfaction. *Journal of Family Practice, 5*(2), 217–222.

Blumer, H. (1966). *Symbolic interactionism.* Englewood Cliffs, NJ: Prentice-Hall.

Bochner, A. P., & Kelly, C. W. (1974). Interpersonal competence: Rationale, philosophy, and implementation of a conceptual framework. *Speech Teacher, 23,* 279–301.

Bostrom, R. N. (1984). *Competence in communication: A multidisciplinary approach.* Beverly Hills, CA: Sage.

Bowman, J. C., & Ruben, B. D. (1986). Patient satisfaction: Critical issues in the implementation and evaluation of patient relations training. *Journal of health care Education and Training, 1*(2), 24–27.

Brislin, R. W. (1981). *Cross-cultural encounters: Face-to-face encounters.* New York: Pergamon.

Cline, R. J. (1983, April). Interpersonal communication skills for enhancing physician–patient relationships. *Maryland State Medical Journal,* 272–278.

Cline, R. J., & Cardosi, J. B. (1983). Interpersonal communication skills for physicians: A rationale for training. *Journal of Communication Therapy, 2*(2), 137–156.

Droste, T. (1988). Quality care: Elusive concept deserves defining. *Hospitals, 62,* 58–59.

Ellingworth, H. W. (1977). Conceptualizing intercultural communication. In B. D. Ruben (Ed.), *Communication yearbook 1* (pp. 89–98). New Brunswick, NJ: Transaction.

Ernstene, A. C. (1957, November 2). Explaining to the patient: A therapeutic tool and professional obligation. *Journal of the American Medical Association, 170,* 1110–1113.

Fine, V. F., & Therrien, M. E. (1977). Empathy in the doctor–patient relationship: Skill training for medical studies. *Journal of Medical Education, 52,* 752.

Furnham, A., & Bichner, S. (1986). *Culture shock: Psychological reactions to unfamiliar environments.* London: Methuen.

Greenfield, S., Kaplan, S., & Ware, J. E. (1985). Expanding patient involvement in care: Effects on patient outcomes. *Annals of Internal Medicine, 102,* 520–528.

Greenfield, S., Kaplan, S., & Ware, J. E. (1986). Expanding patient involvement in care: Effects on blood sugar. *Annals of Internal Medicine, 34*(2), 819A.

Gudykunst, W. B., & Kim, Y. Y. (1984). *Communication with strangers: An approach to intercultural communication.* New York: Random House.

Hall, E. (1959). *The silent language.* Garden City, NY: Anchor Press.

Kaplan, S., Ware, J. E. & Greenfield, S. (1986). Effect of patient attitudes on success of programs designed to expand patient involvement in care. *Clinical Research, 34*(2), 822A.

Kelly, E. W. J. (1979). *Effective interpersonal communication: A manual for skill development.* Washington, DC: University Press of America.

Kim. Y. Y. (1988). *Communication and cross-cultural adaptation.* Clevedon, England: Multilingual Matters.

Kleinman, A. (1980). *Patients and healers in the context of culture: An exploration of the borderland between anthropology, medicine, and psychiatry.* Berkeley, CA: University of California Press.

Korsch, B. M., & Gozzi, E. K. (1968). Gaps in doctor–patient communication: I. Doctor–patient interaction and patient satisfaction. *Pediatrics, 42,* 855–871.

Korsch, B. M., & Negrete, V. F. (1972). Doctor–patient communication. *Scientific American, 227*(2), 66–74.

Kreps, G. L., Hubbard, S. M., & DeVita, V. T. (1988). The role of the physician data query on-line cancer system in health information dissemination. In B. D. Ruben (Ed.), *Information and behavior.* (Vol. 2, pp. 362–374). New Brunswick, NJ: Transaction Books.

Kreps, G. L., Ruben, B. D., Baker, M. W., & Rosenthal, S. (1987). Survey of public knowledge and attitudes about digestive health and diseases: Implications for health education. *Public Health Reports, 102*(3), 270–277.

Kreps, G. L., & Thornton, B. C. (1984). *Health communication.* New York: Longman.

Lane, S. D. (1983). Compliance, satisfaction, and physician-patient communication. In R. N. Bostrom (Ed.), *Communication yearbook 7* (pp. 772–801). Beverly Hills, CA: Sage.

Leebov, W. (1988). *Service excellence: The customer relations strategy for health care.* Chicago: American Hospital Association.

Lewis, R. C. (1983, April). When guests complain. *The Cornell Hotel and Restaurant Association Quarterly,* 23–32.

Mechanic, D. (1982). *Symptoms, illness behavior, and help seeking.* New Brunswick, NJ: Rutgers University Press.

Miller, J. G. (1965). Living systems. *Behavioral Science, 10,* 193–237.

Northouse, P. G., & Northouse, L. L. (1985). *Health communication: A handbook for health professionals.* Englewood Cliffs, NJ: Prentice-Hall.

Physicians for the Twenty-First Century. (1984). Washington, DC: Association of American Medical Colleges.

Ruben, B. D. (1972). General systems theory: An approach to human communication. In R. W. Budd & B. D. Ruben (Eds.), *Approaches to human communication* (pp. 95–118). New York: Spartan.

Ruben, B. D. (1976). Assessing communication competence for intercultural adaptation. *Group and Organization Studies, 1*(2), 334–354.

Ruben, B. D. (1978). Communication and conflict: A system-theoretic perspective. *Quarterly Journal of Speech, 64*(2), 202–210.

Ruben, B. D. (1983a). Intrapersonal, interpersonal and mass communication processes in individual and multi-individual systems. In G. Gumpert & R. Cathcart (Eds.), *Intermedia: Interpersonal communication in a media world* (pp. 110–131). New York: Oxford University Press.

Ruben, B. D. (1983b). A system-theoretic approach to intercultural communication. *International and Intercultural Communication Annual, 10,* 131–145.

Ruben, B. D. (1985a). *The bottomline: A patient relations training program.* Morristown, NJ: Morristown Memorial Hospital.

Ruben, B. D. (1985b). Human communication and cross-cultural effectiveness. In L. A. Samovar & R. E. Porter (Eds.), *Intercultural communication: A reader* (pp. 338–346). Belmont, CA: Wadsworth.

Ruben, B. D. (1986). Public perceptions of digestive health and disease. *Practical Gastroenterology, 10,* 25–42.

Ruben, B. D. (1988a). *Communication and human behavior* (2nd ed.). New York: Macmillan.

Ruben, B. D. (1988b). Communication competence: Applying communication theory. In G. P. Radford & B. D. Ruben (Eds.), *Instructor's manual for communication and human behavior* (pp. 1–12). New York: Macmillan.

Ruben, B. D., & Bowman, J. C. (1986). Patient satisfaction. Critical issues in the theory and design of patient relations training. *Journal of Healthcare Education and Training, 1*(1), 1–5.

Ruben, B. D., & Kealey, D. J. (1979). Behavioral assessment of communication competency and the prediction of cross-cultural adaptation. *International Journal of Intercultural Relations, 3*(1), 1–33.

Ruben, B. D., & Kim, J. Y. (1975). *General systems theory and human communication.* Rochelle Park, NJ: Hayden.

Ruben, B. D., & Ruben, J. M. (1988). *Patient perceptions of quality of care: Survey results.* Unpublished manuscript.

Ruesch, J., & Bateson, G. (1951). *Communication: The social matrix of psychiatry.* New York: Norton.

Selye, H. (1956). *The stress of life.* New York: McGraw-Hill.

Shorter, E. (1985). *Bedside manners: The troubled history of doctors and patients.* New York: Simon & Schuster.

Siegel, B. S. (1986). *Love, medicine and miracles.* New York: Harper & Row.

Sneider, I. (1986). *Patient power: How to have a say during your hospital stay.* White Hall, VA: Betterway Publications.

Spitzberg, B. H., & Cupach, W. R. (1984). *Interpersonal communication competence.* Beverly Hills, CA: Sage.

Steiber, S. R. (1988). How consumers perceive health care quality. *Hospitals.*

Stewart, C., & Cash W. (1985). The health care interview. In C. Stewart & W. Cash (Eds.), *Interviewing: Principles and practices* (pp. 321–255). Dubuque, IA: Wm. C. Brown.

Thayer, L. (1968). *Communication and communication systems.* Homewood, IL: Richard D. Irwin.

Thompson, T. L. (1984). The invisible helping hand: The role of communication in the health and social service professions. *Communication Quarterly, 32*(2), 148–163.

Tuckett, D., Boulton, M., Olson, C., & Williams, A. (1985). *Meetings between experts: An approach to sharing ideas in medical consultations.* London: Tavistock.

Waitzkin, H. (1984). Doctor–patient communication. Clinical implications of social scientific research. *Journal of the American Medical Association, 252*(17), 2441–2446.

Waitzkin, H. B. (1986, August). Research on doctor–patient communication: Implications for practice. *The Internist, 27,* 7–10.

Wertz, D. C., Sorenson, J. R., & Heeren, T. C. (1988). Communication in health professional–lay encounters. In B. D. Ruben (Ed.), *Information and behavior.* (Vol. 2, pp. 329–342). New Brunswick, NJ: Transaction.

West, C. (1984). *Routine complications: Troubles with talk between doctors and patients.* Bloomington, IN: Indiana University Press.

Wiemann, J. M., & Backlund, P. (1980). Current theory and research in communicative competence. *Review of Educational Research, 50,* 185–199.

Woolley, F. R., Kane, R. L., Hughes, C. C., & Wright, D. D. (1978). The effects of doctor–patient communication on satisfaction and outcomes of care. *Social Science and Medicine, 12,* 123–128.

5

Small Group
Communication
in Health Care

Rebecca J. Welch Cline
University of Florida

Small groups are ubiquitous social entities. Pervading the health-care system, small groups enjoin members of a subsystem (e.g., administrators, providers, patients) or function as the interface between levels in the larger system (e.g., administrators and hospital staff). Although the functions of small groups in the health-care system vary, their uses illustrate the interdependence of varied components in health-care delivery, policy formation, health-care administration, health promotion, and research.

Fisher (1980) defined the small group as "three or more people whose . . . behaviors exert a mutual and reciprocal influence on one another" (p. 333). Fisher contended that, to the degree that the communicative behaviors of members are interstructured, a group exists. Thus, unlike collections of people or aggregates, small groups exist by virtue of their social interaction.

Small group communication serves the health-care system in a variety of ways. Small group interaction enjoins and coordinates the efforts of various health-care professionals such that a "health-care team" emerges as a reality. Small group communication itself may serve as a health-care intervention (e.g., self-help groups, counseling groups, therapy groups). Interaction among members of small groups of policymakers, administrators, or change agents may serve as a method to assure a high-quality decision-making process, usually directed toward creating a consensus regarding health policy, the efficacy of a particular medical technology, or the administration of a health-care unit. Or perhaps a health-care agency or regulatory group seeks consensus to facilitate the transfer of research findings into everyday medical practice. In these cases, small group communication is treated as a tool or method for discovery of a "best" solution or assessment. Researchers may rely on small group interaction in the form of focus group discussions as a tool for the discovery of ideas, concepts, or hypotheses to serve as the basis for a health-care research program. Likewise, program planners or change agents may use focus groups for conducting health-related needs assessment or to garner feedback on specific health promotion ideas, messages, or strategies in order to assure better public health through improved health-care and promotion programs.

Across levels of the health-care system, participants in small groups interact for a shared desired outcome, the improved quality of health care. This chapter reviews small group communication in the health-care system and illustrates its varied forms and functions and its often-hidden importance in achieving quality health care. Included in the review are groups involved directly in health care (the health-care team and self-help groups) and groups formed to facilitate policy formation, technology assessment and transfer, and health-care administration (consensus decision-making groups and focus groups).

HEALTH-CARE TEAMS

Increasingly, health-care organizations rely on the potential value of small group communication as they institute a team approach to coordinate holistic health care. This section explores the nature of the health-care team as a small group and emphasizes communication as the essence of "teamness."

The Nature of Health-Care Teams

Although health-care teams may be intradisciplinary, the vast majority of health-care delivery is interdisciplinary (Pettegrew & Logan, 1987). An interdisciplinary health-care team consists of numerous "professionals and semi-professionals with differentiated expertise who work together to provide multiple services needed by a patient" (Gifford, 1983, p. 2). Although the primary care team typically consists of the physician, nurse, social worker, and medical technologist (Thornton, 1977, p. 2), teams may include representatives of psychology, psychiatry, occupational and/or physical therapy, nutrition, pharmacology, dentistry, podiatry, health education, gerontology, and communication

(Gifford, 1983). The interdisciplinary approach is used most often to care for particular patient populations (e.g., geriatric patients, cancer patients, victims of heart attacks).

The term *interdisciplinary health-care team* is used in two strikingly different ways. One view poses the team as a network of professionals often linked only by a shared client or patient. In this case, the concept is structural and emphasizes efforts organized loosely around a client. The second view refers to the team as a small group whose members coordinate their efforts explicitly. This concept is dynamic and emphasizes communication. An example of the second view is the operating room team. Although both approaches recognize the interdependence of efforts in accomplishing a common goal, the goal in the second view is clearly a product of explicit social interaction and, thus, is most relevant to this chapter.

Dowling (1978) defined an "ideal" picture of the team that is explicitly coordinating its efforts toward the satisfaction of specific patients' needs:

> A transitory social system, consisting of a number of persons working together for a defined and mutually accepted goal and according to a mutually accepted program in which each member understands and accepts his/her health care functional contribution to that goal. When used in the health care system, the team has as its goal the satisfaction of specific needs of an individual patient, a family, or a whole community. (p. 8)

Clearly, the essence of "teamness" is small group interaction. Andrus (1975) clarified that essence: "The primary health care team is the intimate, permanent team which has continuing interpersonal relationships among its members and which works toward the goal of seeing that a common group of patients receives comprehensive care" (p. 25). Although networks may evolve through a series of one-to-one links, the development of a formal team requires small group interaction as a means of coordinating care.

The Role of Teams as Small Groups in Health Care

Health care, historically the responsibility of the family, now is often the responsibility of the health-care team. The concept of a formal interdisciplinary health-care team developed in response to changes in the structure of health care. Thus, one small group, the health-care team, often has replaced another small group, the family, in overseeing health care.

With public acceptance of hospitals, health care became institution-alized (Palmer, 1983). Early institutional care treated clients' needs as discrete needs met by different types of providers. Social, diagnostic and treatment, psychological, pharmacological, and spiritual needs were the purview, independently, of social workers, physicians and nurses, psychologists and psychiatrists, and the clergy. The team concept in primary care delivery evolved over the past 35–40 years (Kindig, 1975). As professionals recognized their interdependence and as specialization increased, and the variety of roles and professions in health care grew, the need for coordination of health care became evident (Wise, 1972). In conjunction with a more holistic approach to care, the team concept was welcomed as an effort to use resources more efficiently (Charns, 1976; Goldman, 1982). Today, health-care professionals are trained increasingly to use a team model that emphasizes organizational development and small group processes. The larger health-care system recognizes the principle of nonsumma-tivity at play: "the team is more than a mere addition of the sum of the parts" (Thornton, 1976, p. 3).

Communication and the Health-Care Team

A health-care team's effectiveness is contingent upon its capacity to manage the dynamics of group interaction. Like other groups, the health-care team encounters issues and problems related to leadership, role delineation and negotiation, goal setting, problem solving, conflict, power, authority, trust, and support (Gifford, 1983; Palmer, 1983).

Many of the advantages and disadvantages of a team approach to health care are linked to the team's interactive characteristic. In the-ory, the positive potential of the health-care team includes enhanced understanding of the patient's problems, access to a wider range of expertise, the support of colleagues, reduced stress due to sharing re-sponsibility, enhanced access to care for the patient, a variety of per-spectives, and enhanced motivation based on commitment to the team (Gifford, 1983). These positive outcomes depend on direct interaction among team members. Understanding a variety of views and perspec-tives as well as expert information requires interaction on the task dimension while the socioemotional support of members reduces stress, facilitates task accomplishment, and likely enhances the patient's per-ception of access to technical care and supportiveness as well. To the degree that the team succeeds in providing better care, commitment to the team and to the model of care may be enhanced.

Just as the benefits of a team approach are rooted theoretically in effective group interaction, so too are the potentially negative outcomes. Diffusion of responsibility as the group develops "we-ness" may diminish the quality of care. That "we-ness" may evolve through patterns of interaction that focus unduly on the group as an entity, rather than on their interdependent professional responsibilities (Cline & Cline, 1980). Because numerous professionals "treat" the client, the probability of developing a close, unique relationship may be lessened. Unless the team is well coordinated, patients may feel bombarded by numerous professionals, none of whom provide special support in treatment or in the relationship. Ineffective team meetings may be time consuming and may diminish commitment to the team model and to the team. Intradisciplinary jargon may confuse some and create relational distance among members. Conflicting goals and roles may cause duplication of effort or abandonment of some tasks. Finally, control issues are particularly difficult to manage in health care. Traditionally, the physician has always been "in charge." The physician may have difficulty yielding control, whereas other members may be reluctant to share control.

Observations of actual teams clarify the integral nature of communication in the quality of health care provided. Wise (1972) reported typical communication problems among observed health-care teams and contended that the problems were rooted in a failure to emphasize the communication process in preparing the team members to function as a team. Wise found that some members held "secrets," while some physicians operated independently and failed to share information with other members. Team meetings were hampered by late arrivals, physicians arguing among themselves while leaving other members out, silent team members, and so forth. In short, "power issues, role confusion, and communication gaps added up to difficult and unrewarding team sessions" (Wise, 1972, p. 444). The problem was the failure to "train teams as *teams*," to address issues related to group interaction processes. As team-building and communication consultants intervened to focus on the process in that case, the quality of the health-care delivery by the observed teams improved dramatically.

The Future of Health-Care Teams

Health-care teams offer the *possibility* of more cost-effective, comprehensive, and higher quality health care. For example, one study using a family-oriented health team of physicians, nurses, health aides, and social workers demonstrated that, over time, the patients shifted from an illness orientation to a health orientation. That shift represented more effective use of personnel as patients became less physician dependent and relied increasingly on other professionals (e.g., via nursing counseling, health education, rehabilitation, marriage counseling; Beloff & Korper, 1972). However, insufficient data exist to support the implicit proposition that health care via coordinated health-care teams offers a more effective, efficient, or satisfying model to health care than models relying on less coordination. The health-care team literature repeatedly echoes the theme that more research is needed to provide a test of that proposition.

Clearly, *every* patient receives care from representatives of more than one discipline. Thus, to some degree, a "team" always exists in health care. Professionals may be linked "in name only" or they may pursue explicit coordination with one another. The decision to follow a team model formally rests with the larger health-care organization or system (i.e., the clinic, hospital, or institution). As the team increasingly comes into practice as a model for health care, small group communication becomes a major mechanism for accomplishing health care. Yet, beyond a few case studies, little is known about that communication. Communication researchers need to address questions of how the nature of the team's small group communication is related to the quality of health care provided, job satisfaction, patient satisfaction, and cost of care. Clearly, communication is "a prime focus in the . . . health-care team" and only through communication research can the health-care system discover how to facilitate team delivery of the most effective care (Thornton, 1977, pp. 16–17).

Health-care teams enjoin professional health-care providers in order to improve health-care delivery. Another type of small group involved directly in health-care delivery is the self-help group. In contrast to the health-care team, self-help group members are both helped and become providers of help as the group interaction constitutes the form of health care.

SELF-HELP GROUPS

More than 500,000 self-help groups offer support to people who are coping with crises, role transitions, or problems (Naisbitt, 1982). These systems of individuals, who often share only their particular problem, create an "enduring pattern of continuous or intermittent ties" that can "play a significant part in maintaining the psychological or physical integrity" of their members (Caplan, 1974, p. 7). The nature of self-help groups, their roles in the health-care system, and the place of communication in their mission are explored.

The Nature of Self-Help Groups

Social Support and Health. Growing evidence suggests that exposure to crises or stress is related to the probability of experiencing serious illness (Antonovsky, 1979; Cohen, 1979; Dohrenwend & Dohrenwend, 1974; Rahe & Arthur, 1978; Selye, 1978). At the same time, research indicates that social support can function to buffer or cushion people from the illness-inducing effects of stress (e.g., Dean & Lin, 1977; Kaplan, Cassel, & Gore, 1977). Moreover, social support can ameliorate the effects of an existing illness. For example, the longevity or terminally ill cancer patients can be enhanced by social support (DiMatteo & Hays, 1981).

Social Support and Self-Help Groups. An individual's support net work is "that set of personal contacts through which the individual maintains his [or her] social identity and receives emotional support, material aid and services, and new social contacts" (Walker, MacBride, & Vachon, 1977, p. 35). Dean and Lin (1977) identified the family as the typical principal provider of social support by virtue of the family's emphasis on mutual responsibility, caring, and concern; strong mutual identification; emphasis on the uniqueness of individuals; face-to-face interaction; intimacy; and the provision of support, responsiveness, and security (p. 407). Albrecht and Adelman (1987) clarified the communicative nature of social support: "verbal and nonverbal communication between recipients and providers that reduces uncertainty about the situation, the self, the other, or the relationship and functions to enhance a perception of personal control in one's life" (p. 19).

When our typical first avenues for seeking help, family and friends, and then professional helpers, are unwilling, unavailable, unaffordable, or ineffective, self-help groups offer a viable alternative source of social support. Silverman and Cooperband (1975) clarified the alternative: "Mutual help groups are defined as those organizations that limit their membership to individuals with common problems. The purpose of such organizations is to help the members and others with the same difficulty solve their mutual problems" (p. 13).

Growth and Membership. More than 15 million Americans seek social support through self-help groups (Naisbitt, 1982). According to the popular futurist, John Naisbitt (1982), one of the 10 "megatrends" currently transforming the nature of life in our society is the shift from institutional help to self-help. Naisbitt contended that Americans have become disillusioned with institutional help. Although that disillusionment may account for some of the growth of the self-help movement as an alternative to professional help, changing social structures may make self-help groups a viable alternative to the circle of family and friends as well. (See Cluck & Cline, 1986 for a thorough discussion of the relative advantages of self-help groups.)

Typically, candidates for self-help groups are stigmatized in some fashion (Goffman, 1963). As a result of changing or lost roles or a "spoiling" feature of identity (e.g., obesity, homosexuality), they are trying to cope with social alienation in addition to the personal alienation accompanying a particular problem or predicament (e.g., alcoholism, drug addiction, bereavement, homosexuality, rape, sexual abuse, or obesity). For example, typically both the terminally ill and those experiencing grief are stigmatized and shunned by friends and family (e.g., Parkes, 1970; Perkins, 1981; Stephens, 1972). As a result, social networks are often an exacerbating rather than a healing factor. Family and friends tend to see the individual as "the problem," whereas self-help group members reframe the problem as a more general one in which he or she is a participant (Toch, 1965).

Similarly, professional caregivers may treat the individual's predicament as an illness, a disease, or a defect in perception (e.g., Elbirlik, 1983). A cold and analytic communication climate may result in further social isolation and stigmatization of the individual (Doyle, 1980). Additionally, health-care professionals receive little formal education regarding alcoholism, drug abuse, sexual abuse, terminal illness, homosexuality, bereavement, and other major life crises and problems. As a result, they are likely to approach all problems as illnesses or may see the predicaments as outside of their professional purview. Finally, a lack of communication training may constrain providers' abilities to offer social support.

Relationship of Self-Help Groups to the Larger Health-Care System

Naisbitt (1982) focused on self-help groups as *alternatives* to institutional care. However, the relationship between self-help groups and the larger health-care system is more complex and diverse than Naisbitt implied. Self-help groups *can* function as separate and alternative forms of health care. However, often the groups function explicitly (and always implicitly) as *adjuncts* to or as subsystems comprised of participants in the larger health-care system (e.g., Killilea, 1976).

Self-Help Groups as Alternative Care.   Self-help groups may organize in response to ineffective or unavailable services. For example, the Veterans' Administration organized psychotherapy groups for Vietnam veterans, yet "many vets distrusted not only 'establishment' psychiatric services, but even the private offices of former combat psychiatrists, themselves VVAW members. . . . The VVAW membership opted for rap sessions to fill an unmet need—the need to 'get their heads together' " (Shatan, 1973, p. 641). Similarly, the gay community's dissatisfaction with clinically oriented treatment by nongay mental health professionals led to Gay Growth groups (Killilea, 1976). Other groups spring up to meet needs rejected by the traditional health-care system (e.g., Weight Watchers, groups of smokers trying to quit).

Self-Help Groups as a Subsystem in Traditional Health Care. Self-help groups coordinated their efforts with traditional health-care providers as early as 1905 when "classes" for tuberculosis patients—comprised of weekly meetings of patient groups—were formed in the Boston area (Pratt, 1963). Stichman and Schoenberg (1972) described a program for groups of wives of coronary patients who meet with a professional to share strategies for coping with the husbands' illness and necessary life-style changes. Likewise, the United Ostomy Association coordinates its efforts with traditional providers by providing hospital visitation (with the surgeon's permission) by an ostomate to a person about to undergo ileostomy or colostomy (Lenneberg & Rowbotham, 1970).

In Seattle, Washington, the Washington Association for Sudden Infant Death Study coordinates the management of every case of unexplained infant death. Each case is referred to a pediatric pathologist who performs an autopsy. The report immediately is provided to families who are sent literature and visited by a nurse. Later, parents act as resources to other parents (Pomeroy, 1969).

Recently, researchers discovered that, by having diabetics participate in discussion sessions in which they brainstormed solutions to the problems they anticipated they would face in self-care, the diabetics increased their compliance with their treatment regimen (Pryor & Mengel, 1987). Thus, self-help groups may contribute to health care as an alternative to or in conjunction with traditional care systems.

Communication in Self-Help Groups: Forms and Functions

Although self-help groups vary in the problems that bring members together, groups share certain characteristics. First, most members are stigmatized. Second, as they gather to gain social support, they tend to rely on a set of common principles, including commonality of experience and mutuality of support while developing an informal leadership (Giddan & Austin, 1982; Killilea, 1976). Finally, because the primary function served by self-help groups is that of providing social support, their effectiveness is contingent upon managing group communication processes. Although some types of self-help groups adhere to particular rituals or regimens (e.g., Alcoholics' Anonymous, Weight Watchers), generally groups manage their communication by focusing on creating a particular type of communication climate based on the principle of commonality of experience.

The Form of Communication. The effectiveness of self-help groups appears to be dependent on nurturing a highly cohesive group whose goals are attainable only through communication characterized by reciprocity of self-disclosure, empathic honesty, acceptance, and symmetrical interaction.

Reciprocity of self-disclosure is required for establishing awareness of commonality of experience. In turn, that commonality facilitates group cohesiveness required to achieve the groups' goals. Similarity of experience generates member credibility, contributes to ease of identification, and triggers further reciprocal communication (Cluck & Cline, 1986). Researchers agree that the social support of self-help groups is contingent on similarity of experience (e.g., Silverman & Cooperband, 1975; Walker et al., 1977). For example, Vietnam veterans required the assistance of other Vietnam vets to successfully cope with their unique experience (Shatan, 1973). Members of Compassionate Friends (a self-help group exclusively for bereaved parents) express frustration and anger when others equate the loss of a child with any other loss (Sherman, 1979).

Similarity of experience is argued to account for a lack of hierarchical structure that contrasts with professional psychotherapy groups: "The patterns of communication are from equal to equal rather than from subordinate to superior. . . . Status can be achieved by being a generous giver as well as recipient of aid" (Katz & Bender, 1976, p. 116).

The Functions of Communication. Self-help group members alternate in the roles of empathic listener and discloser. Communication performs two major related functions: identity management, or the process of redefining the self, and the enhancement of perceived control (see Arntson & Droge, 1987, for a discussion of the latter function).

Symbolic interactionist theory (e.g., Manis & Meltzer, 1978) suggests that the self is comprised of roles that are developed and maintained through communication. Members of self-help groups seek to clarify who they are. All are stigmatized. Many have lost roles involuntarily (e.g., through death or divorce). Some have gained new roles (e.g., retirement). Others struggle to replace old roles (e.g., alcoholic, spouse abuser) with new ones. Self-help groups expose new members to role models, provide a safe "stage" for role rehearsal, and permit experienced members further practice. Members share information, gain feedback, and identify behavior changes, all processes that function to enhance members' perceptions of control in their lives.

In contrast to health-care teams and self-help groups, whose functions are directly related to health care delivery, the remaining groups facilitate improved health care in less direct ways through discovery.

CONSENSUS DECISION MAKING
AND SMALL GROUPS IN HEALTH CARE

Consensus in the Health-Care System

The nature of health-care issues magnifies the importance of consensus decision making. The health-care system, both at personal care and policy making levels (e.g., by hospital administrators, health-care agencies) frequently requires decision making "in the face of uncertainty" (Horn & Williamson, 1977, p. 922). In the absence of firm data, health-care providers, health program planners, and policymakers alike are confronted with diagnostic, treatment, educational, and legislative/regulatory decisions. Often, "deferring a decision is not acceptable to the clinical or public health care provider nor to the patient and public" (Kaplan & Farer, 1980, p. 2736). As a result, the health-care system often "decides what is best by the concurrence of judgments of a number of experts in the field" (p. 928).

Groups make decisions via diverse procedures (e.g., negotiation, voting). Evidence suggests that groups that achieve consensus fare better in decision quality.[1] Hirokawa (1982) defined consensus as the "unanimous agreement among group members regarding the group's decision" (p. 407).

Methods of achieving consensus decisions in the health-care system are reviewed here. Participants in consensus decisions may be patients, providers, researchers, policymakers, or a mixture of participants; but the goal is always defining clear actions for improving public health.

---

[1]Consensus decision making enhances objectivity and decision quality when problems are approached systematically and all feasible solutions are considered (Gouran, 1969; Hirokawa, 1982). Also, when the group's goal is the generation of ideas, groups produce more and better ideas than do individuals working alone (Shaw, 1981). Although consensus is not easily achieved (Kerr et al., 1976), research on group interaction finds that the benefits of consensus likely are accomplished through certain features of the group's communication, including greater participation, expression of diverse points of view, and the encouragement of minority opinions and conflict (e.g., Hall, 1971; Maier & Solem, 1952; Nemeth, 1977).

Methods for Achieving Consensus

Three types of consensus achieving procedures are described for managing dilemmas or difficult decisions. Note that these are not recommended for *routine* decisions. Each offers a systematic and exhaustive means of garnering the often diverse and conflicting views of numerous experts in order to facilitate more immediate action (e.g., treating patients most effectively, assigning tasks to a nursing staff, garnering political support for a public health issue). The Delphi and nominal group techniques have been used widely in health care and in other fields. In contrast, the consensus development conference is a method developed by the National Institutes of Health (NIH) to deal specifically with the health-care system.

The Delphi Technique.   A Delphi approach to group consensus usually involves people in three roles. *Decision makers* seek a decision (e.g., hospital administrators, national health policymakers, a health agency). A *planning group* plans, develops, and conducts the procedure. *Experts* are respondents whose judgments are sought.

A Delphi procedure consists of an iterative questioning method. Experts respond in writing to multiple rounds of questionnaires received through the mail. Usually the series begins with a broad question (e.g., asking respondents to generate a list of problems, solutions, objectives, or forecasts). Where appropriate, the experts are provided with a position paper or informative document (e.g., a state-of-the-art review or a series of research abstracts) with the first round. Later rounds of questionnaires may re-ask questions or ask additional questions; after the first round each successive round is designed on the basis of the results of the previous round and features feedback regarding responses on the earlier round. Later findings may be put in quantitative or statistical form. Questionnaire data often are supplemented with interviews to check interpretations. Rounds continue until consensus emerges, sufficient information is generated, or costs are prohibitive.

The Delphi technique has been used in the health-care system for forecasting change, alerting participants to the latest scientific advances, identifying program objectives and strategies, assessing treatment recommendations, and seeking convergence to induce consensus in a larger context. For example, Kaplan and Farer (1980) used the technique to identify a treatment recommendation for people (ages 1–15) possibly infected with drug-resistant tuberculosis bacilli. Loughlin and Moore (1979) obtained consensus regarding the objectives for an academic medical department.

The following example clarifies the function of multiple rounds in achieving consensus. Goodale and Gander (1976) queried 143 chairs of pathology departments in medical schools in the United States and Canada about expected changes in the field. Participants first generated a list of projected changes. The second round provided feedback from the first round and the opportunity to respond again, and asked respondents to suggest the probability that each identified change would occur. Round three included results from round two, the opportunity to reassess probabilities, and asked respondents to project *when* the changes would occur. The final round included data on the projected dates, the opportunity to alter projected dates, and asked if those changes *should* occur as well as what factors would help or hinder the changes. Results were used to develop policies for dealing with anticipated changes.

The Delphi technique permits canvassing a large group of experts spread geographically and without the risk of undue influence by particular individuals. Proponents of the method argue that anonymity of response enhances objectivity, multiple rounds encourage thorough analysis, and independent thinking brings a range of opinions and clarifies the complexity of issues (Loughlin & Moore, 1979). The drawbacks of the method, the lack of socioemotional rewards associated with face-to-face interaction and a lengthy time requirement (at least 2 months), are overcome by the nominal group technique, a method used for similar purposes.

Nominal Group Technique. Developed by Delbecq and Van de Ven (1971), the nominal group technique (NGT) takes its name from the fact that participants are a group "in name only" during some phases of the decision process. Like the Delphi, decision makers, a planning staff, and expert participants are included. The NGT also requires a trained group facilitator. A group sits around a table and responds, in writing, to questions at the facilitator's direction. After writing responses, participants share their ideas singly in round-robin fashion until all ideas are presented. The facilitator records ideas. Next, the group discusses each idea. Finally, independent voting (rank ordering or rating, depending on the nature of the problem or issue) occurs and the group's decision is calculated mathematically by pooling the individual votes (Delbecq, Van de Ven, & Gustafson, 1975).

The NGT has been used with the staffs of health-care facilities (e.g., hospitals or clinics) to identify the most cost-effective actions for improving patient health outcomes (Horn & Williamson, 1977). Trivedi (1982) used the technique to analyze the activities of a nursing staff in a 193-bed short-term general hospital and to compare actual task delegation with hospital policy.

Both the Delphi and NGT generate more ideas than do traditional brainstorming methods (Ulschak, Nathanson, & Gillan, 1981). The nominal group technique takes less time than the Delphi. But the Delphi offers the flexibility of adjusting questions and focal points based on responses. Both methods provide an orderly process for structuring decision making and achieving consensus.

Consensus Development Conferences.   The ultimate goal of the NIH consensus development conference (CDC) is technology transfer, the process of putting scientific findings into everyday clinical practice. Conferences are designed to bring diverse members of the health-care system together (practitioners, consumers, and researchers) to establish a consensus on the safety, efficacy, and appropriateness of using various medical technologies.

Begun in 1977, the conferences have evolved into a formula approach to topics as diverse as the benefits and risks of dental implants, surgical treatment of obesity, breast cancer treatments, childbirth by Caesarean, diets and hyperactivity in children, and total hip joint replacement. Topics are selected according to medical importance (in terms of number of people affected), uncertainty due to a gap between knowledge and practice, and the existence of "sufficient data" for expert scrutiny (Mullan & Jacoby, 1985).

The CDC provides a formal process for identifying and evaluating research discoveries to determine if they are ready for use by the health-care system (e.g., surgical and medical procedures, drugs, devices), identifying and eliminating outmoded and harmful approaches (Kalberer, 1979, p. 3), and alleviating the practice of questionable technologies "in the face of scant information about their health benefits, clinical risks, cost-effectiveness, and societal side-effects" (p. 3).

Consensus development conferences are based on three traditions: the judicial process in which evidence is considered by a jury of peers, the scientific meeting in which experts present their latest findings to colleagues, and the town meeting that provides an open forum for interested and affected parties (Mullan & Jacoby, 1985).

A CDC consists of a 2 1/2- to 3-day meeting of an independent broad-based panel (e.g., basic researchers, clinical practitioners, methodologists, and the public) that considers evidence regarding specified questions. Researchers who represent and advocate strong and often conflicting views present evidence in public sessions. The panel meets in executive sessions to consider evidence and to draft a formal consensus statement. The statement is disseminated immediately in a press conference, is reprinted in medical journals, and is distributed in booklet form to thousands of practitioners, researchers, journalists, libraries, consumer groups, and the public.

The final product of a successful CDC is the translation of research results into the everyday practice of medicine and prevention (Jacoby, 1985). CDCs receive wide coverage in the lay press (Rogal, 1984) and, at their best, set off a chain of events that allows consumers to make more informed decisions about their own health care and prevention needs. For example, the 1984 CDC on high blood cholesterol served as an impetus to heighten the public's concern regarding a major risk factor associated with heart disease. Resulting publicity and lay press coverage triggered public concern; in turn the public sought professionals' help. Many physicians were unprepared to test patients or to interpret those tests and required additional education in order to meet their patients' needs. Since that CDC, cholesterol has become a household word and a matter of public concern. Similarly, the 1986 conference on the health implications of smokeless tobacco, in conjunction with the Surgeon General's Report and other publicity efforts, focused health professionals' and the public's attention on a previously ignored major health issue.

In summary, the quality of health care, and the ability of patients and professionals to make wise health-care decisions, is often rooted in group decision making by a body of experts following a systematic process for guiding members of the health-care system in the face of an otherwise uncertain path.

FOCUS GROUPS

Focus group discussions are a valuable tool in health communication and education for both exploratory research and program planning and evaluation. This section clarifies the nature and uses of focus groups and the integral role of small group communication in using the method successfully.

The Nature of Focus Groups

Basch (1987) described focus groups as "a qualitative research technique used to obtain data about feelings and opinions of small groups of participants about a given problem, experience, service, or other phenomenon" (p. 414). Researchers seek open and in-depth discussion of feelings, motivations, and subjective reactions in an attempt to "experience the experience" and to clarify the "everyday perspectives" of the population being investigated (Calder, 1977, p. 361). Traditionally, focus groups have been associated with marketing research (often as a means of gaining insights into consumers' thinking or reactions to particular products or advertising concepts). However, more recently, focus groups have gained extensive use in health-related research and program planning (Basch, 1987).

A Typical Focus Group. A typical focus group consists of a 1- to 3-hour group discussion with a small group of participants (previously strangers) who are guided by a moderator trained in small group processes (Basch, 1987; Cox, Higginbotham, & Burton, 1976; Levy, 1979; Wells, 1974). The moderator follows a protocol of topics and questions that is designed to elicit group members' responses to particular issues. Transcripts of discussions are developed and analyzed in order to derive insights into the group's "everyday perspectives" on the phenomenon being studied.

Generally, groups are formed to be homogeneous with regard to variables that might influence openness of discussion (e.g., age, gender, ethnicity, social class; NCI, 1984; Wells, 1974). While a diversity of views is sought, homogeneity of group composition is argued to be important in order to explore sensitive topics (e.g., family planning, sexual activity). The critical issue is enhancing openness while reflecting characteristics of the targeted population. For example, Cline and Freeman (1988) conducted focus groups with heterosexual college students regarding AIDS. The researchers formed groups to achieve homogeneity with regard to gender, age, ethnicity, and sexual experience. Among the sexually active, groups were further segmented by whether or not participants (or their partners) used condoms.

Although acquaintances may be more naturally comfortable (Wells, 1974), particularly on conventional topics of conversation, respondents may be less candid with acquaintances than with strangers (i.e., the "stranger-on-the-train phenomenon"), particularly on sensitive issues (e.g., alcohol or drug use, birth control). In addition to not knowing each other, members rarely are informed of the specific topic in advance (NCI, 1984) in order to enhance spontaneity of responses.

In any given study, the number of focus groups needed depends on the number of subgroups being studied, the research aims, cost, and variability of response (Basch, 1987). Typically, a minimum of three or four groups are conducted (Calder, 1977); the guiding principle is to continue groups until largely similar responses are observed.

Uses for Focus Groups

Focus groups are a powerful tool for generating qualitative data. Focus groups permit insight into complicated subject matter, gather in-depth information on many topics in a relatively short time, and allow researchers to clarify responses and to improvise in order to pursue "unexpected but potentially valuable lines of questioning" (Basch, 1987, p. 434).

Approaches. Two primary approaches to focus groups are used in the health arena, the exploratory approach and the phenomenological approach (Calder, 1977). Calder distinguished the two approaches by explaining their differing roles in conducting science. The exploratory approach to focus groups is "prescientific." That is, scientists use focus groups to stimulate their thinking in the early stages of a research program. "The rationale . . . is that considering a problem in terms of everyday explanation will somehow facilitate a subsequent scientific approach" (Calder, 1977, p. 356). In the exploratory approach, focus groups are used to generate scientific constructs, the building blocks of theory, and hypotheses (predictions regarding relationships among constructs). Here, focus groups help scientists to validate their thinking against the everyday experience. Their results serve as the basis for continued research.

In contrast, the phenomenological approach to focus groups attempts to identify points of "intersubjectivity" (general agreement) among a sample representative of a target group (e.g., consumers). The phenomenological approach is intended to help program planners, management, and marketing executives to "get in touch with" targeted segments of the population. Often the participants respond to a specific concept, product, or plan (e.g., physicians' reactions to a cholesterol education approach, teenage girls' reactions to a videotape on breast self-examination). This approach assumes that "reality in the executive suite" may differ drastically from that encountered by patients, physicians, and health-care providers. In this case, focus groups function to bridge the social distance between program planners and users of the program, usually for immediate practical applications.

Specific Uses. Focus groups have been used for a diversity of purposes in the health-care system as well as in marketing research (e.g., Axelrod, 1975a; Basch, 1987; Goldman, 1976; Peterson, 1975). Exploratory uses of focus groups may be the first step in a research program (e.g., Cline & Freeman, 1988) in order to organize the researchers' thinking, identify concepts, and avoid having predispositions influence research outcomes. Focus groups may be used to plan a survey. For example, researchers planning a national survey on public knowledge, attitudes, and behaviors related to breast cancer conducted focus groups with White, Black, and Hispanic men and women in order to identify and formulate key issues. Previously, little information was available on the perceptions and beliefs of men and minority groups. Results were used to formulate hypotheses and to identify language for phrasing questions more clearly and appropriately (NCI, 1984). Kisker (1985) designed a focus group study in order to discover the reasons why teenagers do not practice contraception effectively. Similarly, Heimann-Ratain, Hanson, and Peregoy (1985) sought the participation of adolescents in order to identify perceived needs and interests relative to developing a smoking prevention program.

In contrast to more broad-based exploratory applications, the phenomenological approach uses focus groups to pretest specific existing or planned concepts, messages, public service announcements, or strategies to be used in health care and promotion. Program names, themes, logos, graphics, or photography can be considered (NCI, 1984). Depending on the targeted group, focus groups may be comprised of health-care providers, patients, specific risk groups, or the public at large. For example, a marketing firm recruited a group of cardiologists and internists to respond to the concept of an ancillary nutrition service for their heart patients (focusing on weight loss and cholesterol education and monitoring). A county chapter of the American Heart Association pretested names and logos for a prevention program and discovered desired visual symbols (a heart shape or the county's shape) and avoided confusing program names (NCI, 1984).

In a case where focus groups had an immediate impact on health care, the National Cancer Institute recruited health-care providers, patients, and other professional and personal members of patients' support networks to participate in a study of information needs regarding breast cancer (Office of Cancer Communications, 1982). A flow chart of the sequence of events in the diagnosis and treatment of breast cancer was developed in order to identify decision-making points. Groups of health professionals, physicians, staff nurses, physical therapists, pastoral care workers, and social workers who work with breast cancer patients participated as well as groups of chemotherapy patients and their significant others, women who had undergone breast reconstruction and women with recurrent and advanced disease. Based on the results, the varying information needs of patients and their significant others at each decision-making point were identified. Existing NCI print materials were identified for each decision-making point; where none existed previously, new materials were written. For example, no print materials were previously available on breast reconstruction, recurrent disease, or advanced disease.

Characteristic Communication

A skilled moderator and a well-designed protocol are critical to the success of focus group discussions. The moderator's responsibilities are largely contingent on effective group communication skills. The moderator is responsible for creating a nonthreatening and supportive climate in which respondents feel free to interact, self-disclose freely, and pose conflicting viewpoints. Although one's own self-disclosure may stimulate others' openness, the moderator is faced with eliciting sensitive views without interjecting his or her own views (Levy, 1979). Levy likens the role of moderator to "a conductor, orchestrating an improvisation" (p. 37). The job calls for skill in listening, phrasing open-ended questions, probing responses spontaneously, encouraging conflicting viewpoints, facilitating the group's rapport, controlling impeding group influences (e.g., an overdominating member or a "pseudo-expert"), adapting to the group's responses, pacing the discussion to cover numerous topics, balancing participation, summarizing, and making transitions from topic to topic (Aaker & Day, 1983; Axelrod, 1975b; Basch, 1987; NCI, 1984).

Generally, the protocol is designed with an opening to set the tone, establish ground rules for interaction, and outline the scope of topics to be covered. In order to facilitate in-depth discussion of sensitive topics, the protocol is designed to move from the general to the specific and from nonthreatening topics to more threatening topics as the session progresses. At the same time, the protocol is a guide that permits the moderator to follow up on comments and to probe fruitful responses. A well-planned protocol and a skilled moderator in a conducive environment have been reported to elicit "surprisingly open . . . remarks" on such sensitive topics as "attitudes toward, and use of, contraceptives, deodorants, laxatives, sanitary napkins, liquor, and drugs" (Wells, 1974, pp. 2-144–2-145).

SUMMARY

Small groups are an often hidden but pervasive feature of the health-care system. The types of groups discussed here vary in size, purpose, topic, and the particular manner in which communication functions. But, in all cases, the groups exist for the purpose of improved public health. And, in each case, the mechanism for that mission is group interaction. To the degree that small group interaction is effective, the quality of health-care delivery may be enhanced directly through teams of health-care providers and small groups as health-care interventions (e.g., counseling, therapy, and self-help groups). Likewise, policymakers, administrators, program planners, and researchers in the health-care system rely heavily on the advice, ideas, and opinions of small groups.

Although health-care delivery and related decision making and research rely heavily on small groups, relatively little systematic research exists to test the efficacy of health-care teams, self-help groups, consensus decision methods, and focus groups versus their alternatives. In each case, an array of case studies, subjective participants' reports, and theoretical premises replace thorough testing of assumed benefits. Existing literature focuses on applications of small group communication principles and methods in health-care contexts rather than on investigating the nature, functions, and potentially unique character of that interaction. A clearer understanding of small group processes in the health-care system is needed to clarify the pragmatic as well as theoretical benefits and costs of their applications. Further research may facilitate better small group communication throughout the interdependent components of the system, which, in turn, may mean better health.

REFERENCES

Aaker, D. A., & Day, G. S. (1983). *Marketing research* (2nd ed.). New York: Wiley.

Albrecht, T. L., & Adelman, M. B. (1987). Communicating and social support: A theoretical perspective. In T. L. Albrecht & M. B. Adelman (Eds.), *Communicating social support* (pp. 18–39). Newbury Park, CA: Sage.

Andrus, L. H. (1975). The health care team: Concept and reality. In R. L. Kane (Ed.), *New health practitioners* (pp. 25–40). (NIH Publication No. 75–875). Bethesda, MD: U. S. Department of Health, Education, and Welfare.

Antonovsky, A. (1979). *Health, stress, and coping.* San Francisco: Jossey-Bass.

Arntson, P., & Droge, D. (1987). Social support in self-help groups: The role of communication in enabling perceptions of control. In T. L. Albrecht & M. B. Adelman (Eds.), *Communicating social support* (pp. 148–171). Newbury Park, CA: Sage.

Axelrod, M. D. (1975a). Marketers get an eyeful when focus groups expose products, ideas, images, ad copy, etc. to consumers. *Marketing News, 8,* 6–7.

Axelrod, M. D. (1975b). 10 essentials for good qualitative research. *Marketing News, 8,* 10–11.

Basch, C. E. (1987). Focus group interviews: An underutilized research technique for improving theory and practice in health education. *Health Education Quarterly, 14*(4), 411–448.

Beloff, J. S., & Korper, M. (1972). The health team model and medical care utilization. *Journal of the American Medical Association, 219,* 359–366.

Calder, B. J. (1977). Focus groups and the nature of qualitative marketing research. *Journal of Marketing Research, 14*, 353–364.

Caplan, G. (1974). *Support systems and community health.* New York: Behavioral Publications.

Charns, M. (1976). Breaking the tradition barrier: Managing integration in health care facilities. *Health Care Management Review, 1*, 55–67.

Cline, R. J., & Cline, T. R. (1980). A structural analysis of risky-shift and cautious-shift discussions: The diffusion-of-responsibility theory. *Communication Quarterly, 28*(4), 26–36.

Cline, R. J., & Freeman, K. E. (1988). *Asking the right questions: A qualitative analysis of AIDS in the minds of heterosexual college students.* Paper presented at the International Communication Association, New Orleans, LA.

Cluck, G. G., & Cline, R. J. (1986). The circle of others: Self-help groups for the bereaved. *Communication Quarterly, 34*, 306–325.

Cohen, F. (1979). Personality, stress, and the development of physical illness. In G. C. Stone, F. Cohen, N. E. Adler, & Associates, *Health psychology: A handbook* (pp. 77–111). San Francisco: Jossey-Bass.

Cox, K. K., Higginbotham, J. B., & Burton, J. (1976, January). Applications of focus group interview in marketing. *Journal of Marketing, 40*, 77–80.

Dean, A., & Lin, N. (1977). The stress-buffering role of social support. *The Journal of Nervous and Mental Disease, 165*(6), 403–417.

Delbecq, A. L., & Van de Ven, A. H. (1971). A group process model for problem identification and program planning. *Journal of Applied Behavioral Science, 7*, 466–491.

Delbecq, A. L., Van de Ven, A. H., & Gustafson, D. H. (1975). *Group techniques for program planning.* Glenview, IL: Scott, Foresman.

DiMatteo, M. R., & Hays, R. (1981). Social support and serious illness. In B. H. Gottlieb (Ed.), *Social networks and social support* (pp. 117–148). Beverly Hills: Sage.

Dohrenwend, B. S., & Dohrenwend, B. P. (Eds.). (1974). *Stressful life events: Their nature and effects.* New York: Wiley.

Dowling, T. P. (Ed.). (1978). *Interdisciplinary health care: What it is and how to make it happen.* (Proceedings of the Second National Institute on Interdisciplinary Health Education and Care). Philadelphia: The Pennsylvania College of Podiatric Medicine.

Doyle, P. (1980). *Grief counseling and sudden death.* Springfield, IL: C. C. Thomas.

Elbirlik, K. (1983). The mourning process in group therapy. *International Journal of Group Psychotherapy, 33*(2), 215–227.

Fisher, B. A. (1980). *Small group decision making* (2nd ed.). New York: McGraw-Hill.

Giddan, N. S., & Austin, M. J. (1982). *Peer counseling and self-help groups on campus.* Springfield, IL: Charles C. Thomas.

Gifford, C. J. (1983). *Health team literature: A review and application with implications for communication research.* Paper presented at the Eastern Communication Association, Ocean City, MD.

Goffman, E. (1963). *Stigma.* Englewood Cliffs, NJ: Prentice-Hall.

Goldman, A. E. (1976, January 16). Group depth interviews also have consulting and creative uses. *Marketing News, 9*, 11, 15.

Goldman, H. (1982). Integrating health and mental health services: Historical obstacles and opportunities. *American Journal of Psychiatry, 139*, 616–620.

Goodale, F., & Gander, G. W. (1976). The future of pathology: A Delphi study of pathology department chairmen. *Journal of Medical Education, 51*, 897–903.

Gouran, D. (1969). Variables related to consensus in group discussions of questions of policy. *Speech Monographs, 36*, 387–391.

Hall, J. (1971, November). Decisions, decisions, decisions. *Psychology Today, 5*(6), 51–54, 86, 88.

Heimann-Ratain, G., Hanson, M., & Peregoy, S. M. (1985). The role of focus groups in designing a smoking prevention program. *Journal of School Health, 55,* 13–16.

Hirokawa, R. Y. (1982). Consensus group decision-making, quality of decision, and group satisfaction: An attempt to sort "fact" from "fiction." *Central States Speech Journal, 33,* 407–415.

Horn, S. D., & Williamson, J. W. (1977). Statistical methods for reliability and validity testing: An application to nominal group judgments in health care. *Medical Care, 15,* 922–928.

Jacoby, I. (1985, September). *Technology assessment in health care: Group process and decision theory.* Bethesda, MD: Office of Medical Applications of Research (OMAR), National Institutes of Health. (Mimeo)

Kalberer, J. T., Jr. (1979). *Biomedical consensus development.* Bethesda, MD: Office of Medical Applications of Research (OMAR), National Institutes of Health. (Mimeo)

Kaplan, B. H., Cassel, J. C., & Gore, S. (1977, May). Social support and health. *Medical Care, 15*(5), 47–58.

Kaplan, J. P., & Farer, L. S. (1980). Choice of preventive treatment for isoniazid-resistant tuberculosis infection. *Journal of the American Medical Association, 244,* 2736–2740.

Katz, A. H., & Bender, E. T. (1976). *The strength in us: Self-help groups in the modern world.* New York: New Viewpoints.

Kerr, N., Atkin, R., Stasser, G., Meek, D., Holt, R., & Davis J. (1976). Guilt beyond a reasonable doubt: Effects of concept definition and assigned decision rule on the judgments of mock jurors. *Journal of Personality and Social Psychology, 34,* 282–294.

Killilea, M. (1976). Mutual help organizations: Interpretations in the literature. In G. Caplan & M. Killilea (Eds.), *Support systems and mutual help: Multidisciplinary explorations* (pp. 37–93). New York: Grune & Stratton.

Kindig, D. A. (1975). Interdisciplinary education for primary health care team delivery. *Journal of Medical Education, 50,* 97–110.

Kisker, E. E. (1985). Teenagers talk about sex, pregnancy and contraception. *Family Planning Perspectives, 17,* 83–90.

Lenneberg, E., & Rowbotham, J. L. (1970). Mutual-aid groups for ileostomy patients. *The ileostomy patient* (pp. 74–87). Springfield, IL: Charles C. Thomas.

Levy, S. J. (1979). Focus group interviewing. In J. B. Higginbotham & K. K. Cox (Eds.), *Focus group interviews: A reader* (pp. 34–42). Chicago, IL: American Marketing Association.

Loughlin, K. G., & Moore, L. F. (1979). Using Delphi to achieve congruent objectives and activities in a pediatrics department. *Journal of Medical Education, 54,* 101–106.

Maier, N. R. F., & Solem, A. R. (1952). The contribution of a discussion leader to the quality of group thinking: The effective use of minority opinions. *Human Relations, 5,* 277–288.

Manis, J. G., & Meltzer, B. N. (Eds.). (1978). *Symbolic interaction* (2nd ed.). Boston: Allyn & Bacon.

Mullan, F., & Jacoby, I. (1985, August). The town meeting for technology. *Journal of the American Medical Association, 254,* 1068–1072.

Naisbitt, J. (1982). *Megatrends: Ten new directions transforming our lives.* New York: Warner Books.

National Cancer Institute (1984, January). *Pretesting in health communications.* (NIH Publication No. 84–143). Bethesda, MD: U.S. Department of Health and Human Services.

Nemeth, C. (1977). Interaction between jurors as a function of majority vs. unanimity decision rules. *Journal of Applied Social Psychology, 7,* 38–56.

Office of Cancer Communications (OCC). (1982, September). *Pretest findings on materials* in the breast cancer patient education unit. Bethesda, MD: National Cancer Institute (typewritten).

Palmer, M. H. (1983). *Effective health care teamwork: A process of socialization.* Paper presented at the Eastern Communication Association, Ocean City, MD.

Parkes, C. M. (1970). The first year of bereavement. *Psychiatry, 33,* 444–467.

Perkins, E. (1981). A stranger who cares: A community response to bereavement. In P. F. Pegg (Ed.), *Death and dying: A quality of life* (pp. 174–177). London: Pitman Books.

Peterson, K. I. (1975). The influence of the researcher and his procedures on the validity of group sessions. In E. M. Mazze (Ed.), *1975 combined proceedings* (pp. 146–148). Chicago: American Marketing Association.

Pettegrew, L. S., & Logan, R. (1987). The health care context. In C. R. Berger & S. K. Chaffee (Eds.), *Handbook of communication science* (pp. 675–710). Newbury Park, CA: Sage.

Pomeroy, M. R. (1969). Sudden death syndrome. *American Journal of Nursing, 69,* 1886–1890.

Pratt, J. H. (1963). The tuberculosis class: An experiment in home treatment. In M. Rosenbaum & M. Berger (Eds.), *Group psychotherapy and group function* (pp. 111–122). New York: Basic Books.

Pryor, B., & Mengel, M. C. (1987, Autumn). Communication strategies for improving diabetics' self-care. *Journal of Communication, 37*(4), 24–35.

Rahe, R. H., & Arthur, R. L. (1978). Life change and illness studies. *Journal of Human Stress, 4*(1), 3–15.

Rogal, D. L. (1984, August). *The lay press and the consensus development process.* Bethesda, MD: Office of Medical Applications of Research, National Institutes of Health. (Mimeo)

Selye, H. (1978). *The stress of life* (rev. ed.). New York: McGraw-Hill.

Shatan, C. F. (1973). The grief of soldiers: Vietnam combat veterans self-help movement. *American Journal of Orthopsychiatry, 43,* 640–653.

Shaw, M. E. (1981). *Group dynamics: The psychology of small group behavior* (3rd ed.). New York: McGraw-Hill.

Sherman, B. (1979). Emergence of ideology in a bereaved parents group. In M. A. Lieberman & L. D. Borman (Eds.), *Self-help groups for coping with crisis* (pp. 305–322). San Francisco: Jossey-Bass.

Silverman, P. R., & Cooperband, A. (1975). On widowhood, mutual help and the elderly widow. *Journal of Geriatric Psychiatry, 8*(1), 9–27.

Stephens, S. (1972). *Death comes home.* New York: Morehouse-Burlow.

Stichman, J. A., & Schoenberg, J. (1972). Heart wife counselors. *Omega, 3*(3), 155–161.

Thornton, B. C. (1976). *Communication and health care teams: A multi-methodological approach.* Unpublished doctoral dissertation, University of Utah, Salt Lake City, UT.

Thornton, B. C. (1977). *Communication and health care teams.* Paper presented at the International Communication Association, Berlin, Germany.

Toch, H. (1965). *The social psychology of social movements.* New York: Bobbs-Merrill.

Trivedi, V. M. (1982). Measurement of task delegations among nurses by nominal group process analysis. *Medical Care, 20,* 154–164.

Ulschak, F. L., Nathanson, L., & Gillan, P. G. (1981). *Small group problem solving: An aid to organizational effectiveness.* Reading, MA: Addison-Wesley.

Walker, K. N., MacBride, A., & Vachon, M. L. (1977). Social support networks and the crisis of bereavement. *Social Science and Medicine, 11*(1), 35–41.

Wise, H. (1972). The primary health care team. *Archives of Internal Medicine, 130,* 438–444.

Wells, W. D. (1974). Group interviewing. In R. Ferber (Ed.), *Handbook of marketing research* (pp. 2-133–2-146). New York: McGraw-Hill.

6

Communication in Health-Care Organizations

Eileen Berlin Ray
Cleveland State University

Katherine I. Miller
Michigan State University

It is particularly useful to consider the role of communication in health-care organizations from a systems perspective. The input is the patient (and to some extent, his or her family), the throughput is the health care received while the patient is a member of the organization (which may range from aggressive preventive treatment to palliative care), and the output is the result of that care (the patient gets well and leaves the hospital; the patient's final days are made comfortable and dignified; the patient dies but the family feels positive about the care received, etc.). The components within the health-care organization are all the people who have some impact on the care the patient receives. These may include the custodians who keep the facility sanitary, the person who initially interviews the patient when he or she is admitted, orderlies, pharmacists, nurses, doctors, and administrators. Depending on the type of health-care organization, the nature of the task, and other factors, the degree of interdependency among these components will vary. What is critical is that relevant information can be shared quickly and accurately among those who need it. For example, effective communication from a nurse to the pharmacist regarding type and dosage of medication is critical for patient care. If a mistake is made, the patient's life may be jeopardized. The dyadic relationships can also serve a cybernetic function. They may act to amplify or counteract deviations in the health-care process. A doctor may write a prescription order on a patient's chart. The nurse relays that order to the pharmacist. The pharmacist questions the request so the nurse contacts the doctor for clarification. Each dyadic link provides necessary feedback so that the health care system can make adjustments. Thus, a systems framework provides a useful way to think about the role of communication within a health-care organization context.

Within this framework, it is necessary to consider both the internal and external communication processes and their impact on health-care delivery. To understand the potential effects of the organization–patient and intraorganizational interdependencies, we distinguish between viewing the health-care organization as (a) a *dispenser* of care and, (b) a *cause* of health-care needs for the providers. As a dispenser, the focus is on how the dynamics within the organization enable the health-care providers to meet the needs of its patients in the best possible way. Thus, we can look at communication processes within the organization as they affect patient care. The interface of the providers with the patients, their families, and the community are of particular relevance here. As a cause of health-care needs, the focus shifts from patient care to how the stresses of providing health care influence the health of the providers. Of particular importance here are the stress levels of health-care providers and the negative physical and emotional/mental effects of dysfunctional stress. As Dye (1985) noted, "It is ironic that an organization dedicated to restoring health and promoting well-being often is detrimental to the health and well-being of the people working there" (p. 3).

Obviously, the relationship between the organization as dispenser and as cause is one of interdependence. If the provider's health needs (both physical and emotional) are not met, the quality of patient care will suffer. And if the organization structure is such that providers feel their ability to provide quality care is impeded, their health/attitudes will be negatively affected.

For the organizational purposes of this chapter, our examination of communication in health-care organizations focuses first on the organization as the dispenser of health care and second on the provision of health care as a source of stress for employees of health-care organizations. Both of these issues are considered by examining communication within the organizational context at the interpersonal, work group, organization, and interorganizational levels.

THE ORGANIZATION AS DISPENSER

The goal of any health-care organization, from emergency treatment centers to traditional hospitals, is to provide quality care to its patients. What is considered quality care can be ascertained in a number of ways from a number of perspectives. For physicians, it may be the number of remissions or successful treatments of patients. For nurses, it may be the feeling that they provided care that improved the quality of their patients' lives. For patients and their families, quality includes all of the aforementioned as well as positive interpersonal relationships with the caregivers. Patients who like their health-care providers, feel that they are listened to, are treated kindly, and generally perceive the interpersonal dynamics as positive, tend to be more satisfied with their medical care (e.g., Burgoon et al., 1987; Kreps & Thornton, 1984; Pendleton & Hasler, 1983; Street & Wiemann, 1987). Families typically not competent in the technical aspects of the treatment their family member is receiving, base their impressions on how they are treated by the staff they encounter. They make attributions of good health care if they are shown consideration whenever they are in the health-care setting (Nyquist, Booms, & Hasler, 1989). In addition, patients and families who feel a positive relationship with their health-care providers may be less likely to take legal action against a health-care provider (May, 1985). So although the actual technical care that is dispensed is obviously critical, the relational components of how it is dispensed are also of great importance.

Health-care organizations differ from other types of organizations in many ways. Of particular importance is the nature of the organizational task. Whether it is physical, mental, or a combination health-care facility, the urgency, often life and death, of patient and family needs is great (Thompson, 1986). The information exchange between health-care professionals is critical to ensure quality care for patients and it is the coordination of all relevant people and activities that is essential for successful health-care delivery (Kreps, 1988). It is useful to examine how communication provides this coordination in health-care organizations at the interpersonal, group, organizational structure, and interorganizational levels. A discussion of each follows.

Interpersonal Level

Within the health-care organization, communication at the interpersonal, or dyadic level, may occur between the health-care provider and patient, between two health-care providers (i.e., doctor–nurse, nurse–nurse), or between provider and technician. Chapter 3 provided a thorough review of the research on interpersonal communication between patients and health-care providers, whereas chapter 4 discussed pathological interpersonal health-care relationships. Expanding the system boundaries to the organizational context, however, changes the interdependencies and dynamics of these dyadic relationships. If we conceptualize patient care within a health-care organization as a series of dyadic linkages, a break in any of the links affects the quality of patient care. For example, data collected in the initial patient interview is used to make critical decisions regarding patient care (Barsky et al., 1980; Thompson, 1986). The patient interview has been described as a special type of two-way communication (Mason & Swash, 1975). If the interviewer is not properly trained in question asking as well as interpreting subtle nonverbal cues of the patient, the resulting information will be incomplete or biased and the resulting health care will be less than optimal.

It is this transactional nature of the communication process between the provider and recipient that can act in a deviation counteracting or amplifying manner. The degree of coorientation between the physician and patient is critical for effective health care (Helman, 1985; Mathews, 1983) and may be influenced by the mutual information exchange between the doctor and patient (Argyle, 1983; Lucas, 1985). Feedback is critical for this function to be served. Unfortunately, many times this does not occur. Patients may be unable or unwilling to adequately communicate their medical concerns to the doctor (Friedman & DiMatteo, 1979) and physicians may not probe subtle verbal or nonverbal cues of the patient.

Within the organizational context, the dyadic linkages, beginning with the patient interview and extending to the ties that are enacted to care for that patient can only be successful to the extent that the information gathered and shared at each linkage point is accurate. Feedback at each point is critical to provide the necessary counteracting or amplifying functions. Effective information gathering and exchange is also essential. However, each additional link in the communication chain increases the system's interdependence and opportunity for distortion. Thus, the more dyadic links involved in the patient's care within the organizational context, the greater the chance that some degree of communication breakdown will occur and ultimately affect the patient's care.

Work-Group Level

Chapter 5 provides an in-depth examination of group communication in health care. However, expanding the system boundaries to examine group communication within the organizational context results in greater interdependencies among team members and requires greater coordination and control of communication and activities (Farace, Monge, & Russell, 1977). One example of groups within the organizational context is health-care teams. Health-care teams are particularly prevalent in the care for the terminally ill. These teams are multidisciplinary and typically include a primary physician, a nurse, social workers, patient-care coordinator, an administrator, and the patient or family (Blues & Zerwekh, 1984). Ideally, the health-care team should work in concert and draw on the diverse expertise of its members. The team should serve the necessary deviation amplifying or counteracting function, keeping the system in a state of dynamic homeostasis in meeting the health-care needs of the patient. In this way, changes can be made in the health care provided while maintaining the necessary balance among the team members. However, it is often the team members, as well as the organizational context, that exacerbate, rather than ameliorate, problems (Vachon, 1987).

In addition, health-care teams are expected to work together, ignoring real or imagined differences and egos, for altruistic goals. However, years of academic training, social and cultural factors, and perceptions of statuses assigned to the health-care professions cannot be ignored. In addition, most have been trained to work independently, not interdependently. They often become team members with no advanced communication training or skills in group dynamics and find it difficult to cross traditional professional (Mount & Voyer, 1980) or gender hierarchies (Campbell-Heider & Pollock, 1987). As Mount and Voyer (1980), quoting Rubin, noted:

> It is naive to bring together a highly diverse group of people and expect that, by calling them a team, they will in fact behave as a team. It is ironic indeed to realize that a football team spends 40 hours a week practicing teamwork for the two hours on Sunday afternoon when their team really counts. Teams in organizations seldom spend two hours per year practicing when their ability to function as a team counts 40 hours per week. (p. 466)

In addition to health-care teams, it is critical that work-group members are able to coordinate their activities in a timely fashion within the health-care organization. However, this is often difficult to do. In a study by Ray (1983a), hospital nurses reported several stressors inherent in the organizational context. These included not being treated like a professional, the politics of the hospital, inadequate information from doctors about patients, and dealing with inefficient departments. Conflict with physicians (Gray-Toft, 1980; Vachon, Lyall, & Freeman, 1978) as well as support staff and administration (Yancik, 1984) and limitations of the physical facility (Ray, Nichols, & Perritt, 1987) are also likely to upset the necessary balance among work group members.

Organizational Level

The structure of a health-care organization has a significant impact on its ability to coordinate activities effectively and subsequently dispense adequate health care. It is both the interconnectedness among different aspects of work tasks and the interdependence among units that are critical (Charns & Schaefer, 1983). This interconnectedness and interdependence can only be accomplished through communication (Costello & Pettegrew, 1979; Kreps, 1986).

Several characteristics lead to effective and efficient coordination among interconnected tasks. Coordination must be increased to the extent that the organization's structure separates components of the work that are highly interconnected. This need for coordination is influenced by factors such as task uncertainty, size and interdependence, and influence (Charns & Schaefer, 1983). For example, the greater the task uncertainty, the greater the need for coordination. When uncertainty is low, departments can act in a routine way, with little need for additional coordination. However, when uncertainty is high, coordination becomes critical. A patient suffering from a rare disease or whose condition is quickly deteriorating for no obvious medical reason increases uncertainty and the need for coordination and information exchange among those caring for the patient (Kreps, 1988).

The larger the organization, the greater the need for coordination. The more departments involved in providing the health care, the more complex the coordination becomes. Increases in the number of links in the communication chain result in more complicated control and coordination processes. As Farace et al. (1977) observed, "If messages must pass through the hands of many people for a critical act of coordination, they may become distorted and the coordination effort may fail. If control messages must be broadcast to many individuals in a short time period, no communication mechanism may exist which can do the job" (p. 16).

Interdependence refers to the necessary interrelationships among work units (Charns & Schaefer, 1983). The most common, complex, and difficult to coordinate in health-care organizations is reciprocal interdependence (Thompson, 1967). This occurs when both units affect each other. For example, all of the units involved in the care of a patient are reciprocally interdependent.

Recipricocal interdependence requires both formal and informal communication networks to maximize information exchange and reduce information equivocality. Both of these networks require the support of both the organizational administration and the various units. Reciprocal interdependence can best be conceptualized as reciprocal communication linkages within these networks. This reciprocity can help ensure the accurate and timely exchange of information among these linkages that is critical for successful health care delivery.

Interorganizational Level

At the interorganizational level, coordination among the components of an integrated health-care system becomes particularly crucial. As health-care provision is considered more and more a community problem (see chapter 2 in this book), the ways in which a wide range of health-care organizations can coordinate their efforts will determine the quality of care available to patients. For example, a number of national programs have been instituted to develop community-based systems of health-care provision in which hospitals, medical schools, public health agencies, and home health-care providers attempt to work together in a cohesive program of health education, prevention, and treatment. Thus, understanding the ways communication works to link these interorganizational efforts is essential to effective coordination and health-care provision.

Eisenberg et al. (1985) recently reviewed theory and research on communication linkages in interorganizational systems. As a great deal of the research they reviewed considered health-care organizations (see, e.g., White & Vlasak, 1970), Eisenberg et al.'s taxonomy of interorganizational communication is particularly relevant in the health-care context. They proposed that interorganizational links can involve eitheir information (i.e., symbolic) exchange or material exchange (i.e., the flow of money, goods, and personnel). Both types of exchange are crucial for the most effective interorganizational linkages. For example, an effective community-based cancer control program would require health-care organizations to exchange information about specific patients and specific programs, as well as exchange personnel for training and a wide variety of material necessary for the effective provision of education and treatment. Eisenberg et al. further proposed that interorganizational linkages can involve a personal link (e.g., between physicians from separate hospitals who share information over dinner or at the golf course), a representative link (e.g., between officials at a county health agency and a medical school attempting to coordinate health education efforts in the community), or an institutional link (a link between two organizations that does not specifically involve individuals). Again, the literature clearly suggests that all three of these kinds of links are necessary for effective coordination among organizations. Eisenberg et al. (1985), however, suggested that forging such links can be difficult, particularly among professionals in health-care organizations. As they noted:

> Perceived status distinctions between different kinds of professionals (notably physicians and social service professionals) limit the extent to which personal linkages are formed between members of these two groups (Monge, Farace, Miller, & Eisenberg, 1983). For representative linkages between individuals, the high turnover associated with professionals can impact negatively on the stability of interorganizational systems, since the turnover of key liaison or boundary role occupants can interrupt long-standing patterns of formal and informal information exchange. Particularly in interorganizational networks where linkages are voluntary, personal, and information-oriented, exchange relations which have developed over time are vulnerable to the effects of professional turnover. (pp. 250–251)

THE ORGANIZATION AS CAUSE

It is clear at this point that the nature of communication within health-care organizations has a significant impact on the quality of care received by patients. The literature just reviewed suggests that quality care depends on effective communication within a wide range of interpersonal linkages, effective communication within the work group, and coordination among organizational subsystems and between health-care organizations within a community. Our attention thus far, however, has centered on the effects of communication on the care provided by health-care professionals. The other side of the coin should be considered as well. That is, communication within health-care organizations can have an important impact on the individuals providing the care (i.e., doctors, nurses, administrators, social workers). Most of the literature in this area has considered how the provision of health care can be stressful to individuals and the extent to which health-care professionals are prone to the syndrome that has come to be known as *burnout*. The remainder of this chapter considers how communication within health-care organizations can effect the level of stress and burnout experienced by workers within these organizations. Once again, we consider several system levels within these organizations, although we should remember that these levels are necessarily interdependent.

Interpersonal Level

Burnout has been defined as a wearing down from the chronic emotional pressures of human service work (Pines, Aronson, & Kafry, 1981), and is characterized by physical, emotional, and mental exhaustion (Maslach, 1982; Pines et al., 1981), by a decreasing sense of personal accomplishment (Maslach, 1982), and by a tendency to depersonalize care recipients (Maslach, 1982). The provision of health care almost always requires the establishment of interpersonal relationships between the health-care provider and the recipient. Maslach (1982) has suggested that this interpersonal relationship is the major cause of burnout among all human service workers, health-care professionals included. As she noted "what is unique about burnout is that the stress arises from the social interaction between helper and recipient" (p. 3).

Pines (1982) suggested that the interpersonal relationships between a health-care provider and recipient are unusual in that the care provider always gives—and rarely receives—emotional resources. This relational asymmetry places a great deal of pressure on the care provider to be communicatively competent, and this pressure can ultimately lead to burnout . Thus, it would seem reasonable to suggest that the nature of the interpersonal communication between the health-care provider and care recipient could influence the extent to which the care provider experiences negative outcomes. Lief and Fox (1963) coined the term "detached concern" to describe a necessary condition for medical students in providing quality care. They suggested that avoiding burnout requires health-care providers to feel a true concern for the patient while at the same time maintaining a large share of emotional distance. Miller, Stiff, and Ellis (1988) supported this notion, finding that caregivers in a psychiatric hospital who perceived themselves as most communicatively responsive were those who had high levels of empathic concern for patients but low levels of emotional contagion. Perceived communicative responsiveness, in turn, had a strong effect on the level of burnout experienced by care providers.

Of course, the relationship between caregiver and care recipient is only one of the many interpersonal relationships within a health-care organization. Relationships among caregivers can also have a large impact on the well-being of employees. For example, Marshall (1980) reviewed literature highlighting relationships with doctors as a potential source of stress for many nurses. She noted that "the traditional role segregation between the responsible diagnosing and treating doctor and the caring nurse is not easily maintained even if both parties agree with its underlying justice" (p. 32). Relationships with family members can also be stressful to caregivers in that "they represent a third party with their own separate attribution of meanings, reactions, and needs for support" (Marshall, 1980, p. 31). Perhaps the most important single relationship beyond the caregiver–care recipient relationship, however, is between the caregiver and his or her supervisor.

A number of writers have pointed to the importance of support from the supervisor in reducing job stress and burnout, particularly in caregiving organizations (see Ray, 1987, for a review of this literature). The communicative support of a supervisor can be useful in a number of ways. First, a supportive supervisor can serve to reduce the level of ambiguity a health-care professional feels about his or her role. Informational support of this kind—particularly providing workers with an opportunity to participate in the decision-making process—is crucial, for role ambiguity has been found to be a major contributor to stress and burnout in workers in general (Kahn, 1978) and in health professionals in particular (Miller, Ellis, Zook, & Lyles, 1988). A supportive supervisor can also provide emotional support by allowing the care provider to vent feelings and by letting the stressed worker know that he or she is not alone. Marshall (1980) suggested that staff meetings—in addition to providing informational support—can supply needed emotional support. "Nurses should have the opportunity to express and share their reactions to their work in regular staff meetings and . . . training should be given to help them understand and cope with anxiety about death and dying" (p. 53).

Work-Group Level

The work group within a health-care organization can serve both as a source of stress and as an important coping mechanism for individuals suffering from stress and burnout. Support from co-workers has long been noted as an important buffer against workplace stressors. It is assumed that co-workers are in an optimal position to provide support, as they have the greatest understanding of the workplace and its inherent stressors (House, 1981; Ray, 1987). Especially in health-care organizations, friends and families may not have sufficient understanding of the workplace context to provide the emotional and informational support necessary for effective coping. However, communication with co-workers can be a double-edged sword. Adelman's (1986) investigation of the "contagion effect" among nurses suggests that the same communication behavior that can serve the useful purpose of venting and sharing frustrations can also lead health-care providers to higher levels of stress as they vicariously experience the stresses of their co-workers as well.

Research supports the importance of work-group linkages as both a positive and negative factor in the lives of health-care employees. A survey of 1,000 nurses (Steffen, 1980) found that although relationships within the work group were the second greatest source of satisfaction at work ("being part of a skilled team" and "peer recognition and support" p. 46), these relationships were also the second greatest source of stress: problems with other nurses ("the continuously competitive atmosphere, along with the lack of comraderie" p. 51) and problems with physicians and supervisors. Likewise, Ray (1983a) found interpersonal relationships between nurses and others in a hospital to be highly stressful. However, Nievaard (1987) found that improved communication among nurses in a Dutch hospital did not significantly effect their attitudes toward patients. Rather, it was problems with the doctors and hospital administration that were positively related to negative attitudes toward patients.

Organizational Level

At the organizational level, the structure of ties among health-care providers appears to affect their ability to cope with the stress inherent in their job and buffer ill health. It is these resulting networks that can impede or enhance the amount of support perceived by providers.

Support is inherently communicative in nature. According to Albrecht and Adelman (1984), support is "the way in which communication behaviors tie an individual to his or her social environment and functions to enable the individual to positively relate to that environment" (p. 4). The communication of support within health-care organizations is developed and maintained through the ongoing, regular interactions among its members (Wellman, 1981). The degree of availability and accessibility of support largely results from the structure of ties organization members have with each other (Gottlieb, 1981). As noted by House (1981), "Flows of social support occur primarily in the context of relatively stable social relationships rather than fleeting interactions among strangers" (p. 29). Of particular importance is the health-care provider's location in the informal communication network as a mediator of negative health outcomes. For example, Anderson and Gray-Toft (1982) found nurses on the day shift with high stress and burnout were located in the center of the support network, whereas evening and night-shift nurses were not. Ray (1983b) found that nurses in a children's hospital who were integrated in their work unit reported less burnout but no less stress than those less integrated. These findings were replicated by Dye (1985) with a sample of intensive care hospital nurses.

However, it is important to recognize that these network ties may act to increase, rather than decrease, stress and burnout. If the content of the ongoing communication is negative, interaction may act in a deviation amplifying manner, increasing the provider's negative affect. This has been referred to as the "contagion effect" (Adelman, 1986; Cherniss, 1980; Ray, 1983b) or reverse buffering (Beehr, 1985). The resulting stress and burnout then must be counteracted with positively valenced messages, often introduced through formal organizational-level interventions (Edelwich, 1980). In addition to message content, research in nonhealth related organizations suggests that network characteristics such as the degree of reciprocity, multiplexity, and strength of communication ties are also negatively related to stress and burnout (Ray, 1986).

Interorganizational Level

The importance of links between organizations for the effective delivery of coordinated health care was discussed earlier. In establishing these interorganizational linkages, and in dealing with the consumers of health care, many health providers find themselves on the "edges" of organizations. Although they are officially affiliated with a particular hospital, office, or health agency, a majority of these individuals' time is spent interacting with outsiders such as patients, families, representatives of other health-care organizations, and government and regulatory agency officials. Clearly, as noted earlier, the quality of these extra-organizational linkages will impact the extent to which it is possible to deliver high quality care. In addition, however, the very process of spanning organizational boundaries can cause extensive stress for the individual employee or health-care provider.

The term *boundary spanner* was coined by Adams (1980) to describe an organizational role in which an individual serves in some way to functionally relate an organization to its environment. Adams noted a number of boundary activities these individuals engage in: (a) transacting organizational inputs and outputs, (b) filtering inputs and outputs, (c) searching for and collecting information, (d) representing the organization, and (e) buffering the organization from external threats. In a health-care organization, boundary-spanning activities would include a wide range of contact with patients and families, supply procurement, establishing and maintaining contacts with other health-care organizations, dealing with insurance agencies, and so on. In short, the very nature of a health-care organization requires extensive boundary spanning activities by a wide range of organizational employees.

Boundary-spanning activities can often be stressful for organizational employees. Adams (1976, 1980) noted that buffering an organization can lead to role conflict, stress, and tension for the boundary spanner in several ways. First, the boundary spanner can experience tension from trying to balance the needs of the organization with the needs of the "outsiders" with whom transactions are taking place. This stress is particularly crucial for individuals in public relations roles, for Adams (1980) noted that "giving the impression to outsiders that their voice is being heard and given weight conflicts with the ethical principle that one should be truthful" (p. 350). Adams (1980) also noted a second source of stress for the boundary spanner: "the frequent hostility of outsiders, especially members of 'activist' groups, attempting to induce change in the organization" (p. 350).

More specific to the health-care context, however, is the specific boundary-spanning activity of contact with patients and their families. Literature on caregivers has repeatedly noted the detrimental effects of large caseloads on the psychological and physical health of human service personnel (Daley, 1979; Maslach & Pines, 1977; Pines & Maslach, 1978). These researchers note that constant interaction with individuals in need of help can be extremely stressful, especially when there is little positive feedback received from the care recipient and when there seems little hope that the level of contact will be reduced. This problem is particularly acute in chronically understaffed health fields such as nursing (Jacobson & McGrath, 1983).

SUMMARY

We noted at the beginning of this chapter that the systems perspective was particularly crucial for a consideration of communication in health-care organizations. The issues we have reviewed in this chapter clarify this point by highlighting the crucial interdependence among health-care providers in a variety of organizational roles, their patients and the patients' families, and the larger community environment in which the health-care organization exists. Clearly, providing quality health care requires coordination at all levels of the organizational system— coordination between the health-care provider and recipient, coordination among health-care team members, coordination among disparate departments within the health-care organizations, and interorganizational coordination among community agencies. This coordinated effort can pay high dividends in terms of the quality of care received by the patient. Unfortunately, the provision of care can also mean high costs for the professional health-care provider in terms of the stress and burnout associated with the caregiving role, although clear role definitions and social support from within the organization can serve to lessen this risk. It is only through an increased understanding of the interdependence of health-care providers and their patients within the health-care organization that we can improve the quality of life for both the caregiver and the care recipient.

REFERENCES

Adams, J. S. (1976). The structure and dynamics of behavior in organization boundary roles. In M. D. Dunnette (Ed.), *Handbook of industrial and organizational psychology* (pp. 1175–1199). Chicago: Rand McNally.

Adams, J. S. (1980). Interorganizational processes and organization boundary activities. *Research in Organizational Behavior, 2,* 321–355.

Adelman, M. B. (1986). *The contagion effect: A study on stress and the provision of support.* Unpublished doctoral dissertation, University of Washington, Seattle, WA.

Albrecht, T. L., & Adelman, M. B. (1984). Social support and life stress: New directions for communication research. *Human Communication Research, 11,* 3–32.

Anderson, J. G. & Gray-Toft, P. A. (1982). *Stress, burnout, and turnover among health professionals: A social network approach.* Paper presented at the annual meeting of the International Sociological Association, Mexico City.

Argyle, M. (1983). Doctor–patient skills. In D. Pendleton & J. Hasler (Eds.), *Doctor–patient communication* (pp. 57–74). London: Academic Press.

Barsky, A. J., Kazis, L. E., Freiden, R. B., Goroll, A. H., Hatem, C. J., & Lawrence, R. S. (1980). Evaluating the interview in primary care medicine. *Social Science and Medicine, 14A,* 653.

Beehr, T. A. (1985). The role of social support in coping with organizational stress. In T. A. Beehr & R. S. Bhagat (Eds.), *Human stress and cognition in organizations: An integrated perspective* (pp. 375–398). New York: Wiley.

Blues, A. G., & Zerwekh, J. V. (1984). *Hospice and palliative nursing care.* Orlando, FL: Grune & Stratton.

Burgoon, J. K., Pfau, M., Parrott, R., Birk, T., Coker, R., & Burgoon, M. (1987). Relational communication, satisfaction, compliance-gaining strategies, and compliance in communication between physicians and patients. *Communication Monographs, 54,* 307–324.

Campbell-Heider, N., & Pollock, D. (1987). Barriers to physician–nurse collegiality: An anthropological perspective. *Social Science and Medicine, 25*(5), 421–425.

Charns, M. P., & Schaefer, M. J. (1983). *Health care organizations.* Englewood Cliffs, NJ: Prentice-Hall.

Cherniss, C. (1980). *Staff burnout: Job stress in the social services.* Beverly Hills, CA: Sage.

Costello, D., & Pettegrew, L. (1979). Health communication theory and research: An overview of health organizations. In D. Nimmo (Ed.), *Communication yearbook 3* (pp. 607–623). New Brunswick, NJ: Transaction-International Communication Association.

Daley;, M. R. (1979). Preventing worker burnout in child welfare. *Child Welfare, 58,* 443–450.

Dye, F. W. (1985). *Supportive communication networks and job stress: A study of intensive care nurses.* Unpublished master's thesis, University of Kentucky, Lexington, KY.

Edelwich, J. (1980). *Burn-out: Stages of disillusionment in the helping professions.* New York: Human Sciences Press.

Eisenberg, E. M., Farace, R. V., Monge, P. R., Bettinghaus, E. P., Kurchner-Hawkins, R., Miller, K. I., & White, L. L. (1985). Communication linkages in interorganizational systems: Review and synthesis. In B. Dervin & M. J. Voigt (Eds.), *Advances in communication science* (Vol. 6, pp. 231–261). Norwood, NJ: Ablex.

Farace, R. V., Monge, P. R., & Russell, H. (1977). *Communicating and organizing.* Reading, MA: Addison-Wesley.

Friedman, H. S., & DiMatteo, M. R. (1979). Health care as an interpersonal process. *Journal of Social Issues, 35,* 82–89.

Gottlieb, B. H. (1981). Social networks and social support in community health. In B. H. Gottlieb (Ed.), *Social networks and social support* (pp. 11–42). Beverly Hills CA: Sage.

Gray-Toft, P. (1980). Effectiveness of a counseling support program for hospice nurses. *Journal of Counseling Psychology, 27*(4), 346–354.

Helman, C. G. (1985). Communication in primary care: The role of patient and practitioner explanatory models. *Social Science and Medicine, 20*(9), 923–931.

House, J. S. (1981). *Work stress and social support.* Reading, MA: Addison-Wesley.

Jacobson, S. F., & McGrath, H. M. (Eds.). (1983). *Nurses under stress.* New York: Wiley.

Kahn, R. (1978). Job burnout: Prevention and remedies. *Public Welfare, 36*(2), 61–63.

Kreps, G. (1986). *Organizational communication: Theory and practice.* White Plains, NY: Longman.

Kreps, G. (1988). The pervasive role of information in health and health care: Implications for health communication policy. In J. Anderson (Ed.), *Communication yearbook 11* (pp. 238–276). Menlo Park, CA: Sage.

Kreps, G., & Thornton, B. (1984). *Health communication.* New York: Longman.

Lief, H. I., & Fox, R. C. (1963). Training for "detached concern" in medical students. In H. I. Lief, V. F. Lief, & N. R. Lief (Eds.), *The psychological basis of medical practice* (pp. 12–35). New York: Harper & Row.

Lucas, I. R. (1985, August). *The effects of initial interaction on uncertainty, rapport, and interpersonal attraction.* Paper presented at the Summer Conference on Health Communication, Evanston, IL.

Marshall, J. (1980). Stress amongst nurses. In C. L. Cooper & J. Marshall (Eds.), *White collar and professional stress* (pp. 19–59). New York: Wiley.

Maslach, C. (1982). *Burnout: The cost of caring.* Englewood Cliffs, NJ: Prentice-Hall.

Maslach, C., & Pines, A. (1977). The burn-out syndrome in the day care setting. *Child Care Quarterly, 6,* 100–113.

Mason, S., & Swash, M. (1975). *Hutchinson's clinical methods* (17th ed.). London: Bailliere Tindall.

Mathews, J. J. (1983). The communication process in clinical settings. *Social Science and Medicine, 17,* 1371.

May, M. L. (1985, August). *Patients and doctors in conflict: The nature of patients' complaints and what they do about them.* Paper presented at the Summer Conference on Health Communication, Evanston, IL.

Miller, K. I., Ellis, B. H., Zook, E. G., & Lyles, J. S. (1988). *An integrated model of communication, stress, and burnout in the workplace.* Unpublished manuscript, Department of Communication, Michigan State University, East Lansing.

Miller, K. I., Stiff, J. B., & Ellis, B. H. (1988). Communication and empathy as precursors to burnout among human service workers. *Communication Monographs, 55,* 250–265.

Monge, P. R., Farace, R. V., Miller, K. I., & Eisenberg, E. M. (1983, May). *Life cycle changes in interorganizational information networks.* Paper presented at the annual meeting of the International Communication Association, Dallas, TX.

Mount, B., & Voyer, J. (1980). Staff stress in palliative/hospice care. In I. Ajemian & B. Mount (Eds.), *The RVH manual on palliative/hospice care* (pp. 457–488). New York: The Free Press.

Nievaard, A. C. (1987). Communication climate and patient care: Causes and effects of nurses' attitudes to patients. *Social Science and Medicine, 24*(9), 777–784.

Nyquist, J. D., Booms, B. H., & Halser, J. (1989). *Communication behaviors for enhancing family and resident satisfaction in nursing homes.* Paper presented at the annual meeting of the Western Speech Communication Association, Spokane, WA.

Pendleton, D., & Hasler, J. (1983). *Doctor–patient communication.* London: Academic Press.

Pines, A. M. (1982). Helpers' motivation and the burnout syndrome. In T. A. Wills (Ed.), *Basic processes in helping relationships* (pp. 453–475). New York: Academic Press.

Pines, A. M., Aronson, E., & Kafry, D. (1981). *Burnout: From tedium to personal growth.* New York: The Free Press.

Pines, A. M., & Maslach. C. (1978). Characteristics of staff burnout in mental health settings. *Hospital and Community Psychiatry, 29,* 233–237.

Ray, E. B. (1983a) Identifying job stress in a human service organization. *Journal of Applied Communication Research, 11,* 109–119.

Ray, E. B. (1983b). Job burnout from a communication perspective. In R. N. Bostrom (Ed.), *Communication yearbook 7* (pp. 738–755). Beverly Hills, CA: Sage.

Ray, E. B. (1986). *Communication network roles as mediators of job stress and burnout: Case studies of two organizations.* Paper presented at the annual meeting of the Speech Communication Association, Chicago, IL.

Ray, E. B. (1987). Support relationships and occupational stress in the workplace. In T. L. Albrecht, M. B. Adelman, & Associates, *Communicating social support* (pp. 172–191). Newbury Park, CA: Sage.

Ray, E. B., Nichols, M. R., & Perritt, L. J. (1987). A model of job stress and burnout. *The Hospice Journal, 3*(2/3), 3–28.

Steffen, S. (1980). Perceptions of stress: 1800 nurses tell their stories. In K. Claus & J. Bailey (Eds.), *Living with stress and promoting well-being* (pp. 38–58). St. Louis: C. V. Mosby.

Street, R. L., Jr., & Wiemann, J. M. (1987). Patient satisfaction with physicians' interpersonal involvement, expressiveness, and dominance. In M. McLaughlin (Ed.), *Communication yearbook 10* (pp. 591–612). Newbury Park: Sage.

Thompson, J. D. (1967). *Organizations in action.* New York: McGraw-Hill.

Thompson. T. L. (1986). *Communication for health professionals.* New York: Harper & Row.

Vachon, M. L. S. (1987). Team stress in palliative/hospice care. *The Hospice Journal, 3*(2/3), 75–103.

Vachon, M. L. S., Lyall, W. A. L., & Freeman, S. J. J. (1978). Measurement and management of stress in health professionals working with advanced cancer patients. *Death Education, 1,* 365–375.

Wellman, B. (1981). Applying network analysis to the study of support. In B. H. Gottlieb (Ed.), *Social networks and social support* (pp. 171–200). Beverly Hills, CA: Sage.

White, P. E., & Vlasak, G. J. (Eds.). (1970). *Interorganizational research in health.* Baltimore, MD: Department of Behavioral Sciences, Johns Hopkins University.

Yancik, R. (1984). Coping with hospice work stress. *Journal of Psycho-social Oncology, 2*(2), 19–35.

III

COMMUNICATION AND PUBLIC HEALTH: MASS MEDIA AND EDUCATION ISSUES

7

Health Images
in the Mass Media

Kimberly A. Neuendorf
Cleveland State University

The various institutions we call *mass media* have in common two principal characteristics. The "media" component indicates that some mechanical or electronic device(s) are interposed between the source of the message and the receiver. The "mass" component does not mean that there are many receivers, but rather that the many diverse receivers are undifferentiated in the source's message—that the message is created for all (or at least all in the target audience of the particular media outlet).

The latter is an important consideration in the process of health communication via mass media. The message is and must be palatable to one and all, and tailored for no one in particular. This is a clear divergence from the goals of face-to-face health communication events, such as those of doctor–patient interaction, or of public health campaigns involving specialized targeting, described in the chapters by Brown and Einseidel and by Donohew.

This is not to say that individuals are not affected by mass mediated messages in distinctly individual ways. Clearly, individual social and psychological differences mediate the way in which information and entertainment content affect the receiver of mass messages. Social learning theory has given mass communication scholars a framework by which to analyze such effects. Bandura (1969, 1971; Bandura & Walters, 1963) has articulated social learning theory's provision that behaviors can, and most likely will, be learned by simply observing others and subsequently imitating (modeling) their behaviors in an appropriate context. This modeling may occur with a media personality as well as a real-life model.

Modeling effects are greater in certain instances. When alternative models are few, when reinforcement is demonstrated, and when the model is similar in manifest characteristics to the receiver or to the type of individual the receiver respects, effects are maximized. Subsequent sections of this chapter explore examples of topic areas in which social learning may occur, but I note at this point the relative paucity of real-life "alternative models" in the health communication context. Admonishing physicians to take note of the constellation of influences their patients are exposed to outside of the doctor's office, Sandman (1976) noted:

> The typical American visits a doctor several times a year. The same American reads a medical article in a newspaper or magazine several times a month; he or she watches a TV show featuring a medical problem several times a week, and may well encounter medical advertising several times a day. The impact of this constant exposure is profound. . . . Inevitably . . . [how much your patients know about medicine and health] depend[s] more on the content of the media than on the conduct of your practice. (p. 378)

Recognizing the pivotal role of *television* in "socializing individuals and stabilizing lifestyles," Gerbner, Morgan, and Signorielli (1982) also noted that "[t]he success or failure of educational and informational [health] campaigns depends largely on the broader cultural context into which they are injected" (p. 291). This constellation of influences may be seen in Fig. 7.1, which indicates the main informational and influential links surrounding the individual. The individual is exposed to entertainment messages coming from television and many other media (Link 1), news and documentary (i.e., "factual") information coming from print and other media (including TV; Link 3), direct contact with health professionals in health contexts (Link 10), and other individuals in one's home and work environments (Link 11). Not immediately tied to the individual is the set of professional organizations associated with health (e.g., AMA), which is connected to the individual largely through the groups' influence on entertainment and news media (Links 7 and 8).

Links 5 and 6 show the occasional but important direct link between individual health professionals and media sources (e.g., when a physician serves as a consultant to a television series). Links 2 and 4 remind us that health professionals are people too, and not entirely immune to entertainment media effects, and certainly regularly exposed to factual

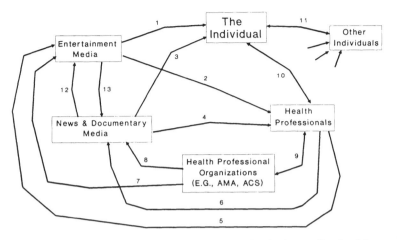

FIG. 7.1. Constellation of influence for the individual regarding health.

information via professional periodicals. Link 9 establishes the connection between professional organizations and their constituencies. Finally, Links 12 and 13 acknowledge the mutual influence of entertainment and news media institutions on one another. Whereas Link 13 again simply reminds us that newspeople are individuals who may be affected by the numerous entertainment images they are exposed to, Link 12 has as its base many examples of news reports of "real-life" health issues influencing entertainment writers' selection of topics (e.g., when soap opera writers covered toxic shock syndrome several years ago as a "public service").

Clearly, other links in the model are possible, as are other components. For example, Gandy (1981) noted the additional component of an "information subsidy" by "government and bureaucracy providers," that impart information directly to consumers and to the entertainment and news media. I would hold that in the health arena much of this influence is felt through the actions of the health professional organizations, operating via mass media; indeed, Gandy's primary example involves the American Cancer Society. However, his point regarding government influence in the system is noteworthy.

Arrows of influence in the model are mostly shown as one way. This is not to indicate a lack of mutuality of influence, but rather to show the dominant influence of one direction. An example of how Links 2 and 4 could flow in the opposite direction would be Williams' (1982) prediction of a "Satellite Health Service," providing two-way medical telecommunications to remote locations. This is presently technically feasible and has been occurring in a small way (e.g., Boston's Logan

Airport's video link with Massachusetts General Hospital; Williams, 1982, p. 177) as the medical profession continues to reach out for the technology of the media.

Not specified in this model is an important component—that of advertising. It is an integral part of both news and entertainment media content. Prior to 1977, "health advertising" was limited to ads for drugs and other health aids; doctors and health institutions did not advertise. In 1977, a Supreme Court decision struck down the AMA's self-imposed prohibition against advertising, and we now see increasing acceptance of self-promotion by health professionals. Indeed, 1985 saw a 40% increase over 1984 in the amount of health-care TV advertising in the United States ("Health-care TV ads continue to grow at sizzling pace," 1986). In 1983 the Television and Radio Codes of the National Association of Broadcasters (NAB), which for many years regulated the specifics of advertising of medical products on TV and radio,[1] were struck down in a Justice Department ruling, which held that they violated antitrust statutes. With this looser environment for health-related persuasive messages has also come a trend in selling nonhealth-related products and services with promises of nutritional value and healthfulness.[2]

For clarity's sake, advertising is not specified in Fig. 7.1 as a separate component, but is treated as part of the entertainment media and news media content. Its source of influence is also not clearly shown—manufacturers of health products; this begins to create another constellation of influences, those with economic power as opposed to informational influence. Given advertising's similarity in form and intent to media campaigns for health issues (see chapter 9, this volume), it is treated in this chapter only when there is a topical need for its discussion, as in the case of the existent literature on alcohol advertising.

It must be noted, as well, that health-related advertising is highly contextualized—that is, its placement is carefully planned to capitalize

---

[1]The NAB Television Code included a requirement that cereal spots aimed at children include a "balanced breakfast" disclaimer. Also included were entertainment programming cautions against gratuitous drug, alcohol, and tobacco abuse.

[2]Kalish (1987) noted such unlikely "healthy" foods as Pringle's potato chips (touting a lower fat content) and McDonalds burgers and fries (in an ad cited by three states' attorney generals as "deceptive"). Neuendorf and Pearlman (1988) have identified "good food" appeals in magazine ads for liqueurs, which have led to teen respondents' perceptions that the products are healthful. Manoff (1986), showing concern for the "propriety" of nutritional health claims in advertising, cited numerous cases in which telling less-than-all has been quite misleading (e.g., in stating that Tofutti is free of lactose and cholesterol, but failing to note that it is higher in calories than ice cream, with 14% fat).

on consumers' conceptual predispositions as they watch, for example, the series of Sunday health programs on the Lifetime cable network, into which are embedded ads with amazing specificity and assumptions of prior medical knowledge. A 1970's analysis of "Marcus Welby, M.D.," found 19 out of 68 TV spots to be for health products, and 28 more to be for food or cosmetics (Real, 1977).

In the following subsections, news and entertainment are dealt with separately in overviews. Then, seven different specific content areas, each of which has received substantial attention in the social scientific literature, are explored: Nutrition and body image, mental illness, substance use and abuse, aging, sexual behaviors, health professional roles, and therapeutic TV. In each case, the emphasis is on entertainment media influence on the individual, with occasional reference to news and documentary media, and with reference to advertising inter jected as appropriate. Entertainment television has received the lion's share of social scientific study, and that is reflected as well.

AN OVERVIEW OF NEWS MEDIA INFLUENCE (LINKS 3 AND 4)

In a review of research on the content of and preferences for health news, Simpkins and Brenner (1984) noted wide interest in health news, continuing over a 25-year period. In a study by Kreighbaum (1959, cited in Simpkins & Brenner, 1984), 40% of the respondents indicated they read *all* medicine and health articles in their daily newspaper. Health news interest seems to be greater among women and higher income individuals, a trend we see continuing in Lifetime's overt plan to capture a female audience with a heavy health emphasis.

For all the interest, coverage of health-related topics has garnered stiff criticism from scientists and health professionals alike (Fisher, Gandy, & Janus, 1981; Freimuth, Greenberg, DeWitt, & Romano, 1984; Whelan, 1987). The fact that the reporting of health news has most often fallen to media professionals, not health professionals, has created a message environment in which only the sensational survives. Whelan (1987) noted a dozen or more much-publicized hypothetical causes of death that have been given premature mortality estimates of near *zero* by the American Council on Science and Health. For example, risk of death due to radiation exposure at Three Mile Island was equivalent to the risk of crossing the street five times, yet Three Mile Island's coverage was immense.

Studies have found consistent evidence of an agenda-setting function of news information in general. The cornerstone of this theoretic approach is that although media may not have the power to determine *what* people think, they can and do determine what people think *about*.

Hence, the amount of press coverage an issue receives will be related to the importance placed on that issue by individuals in the society, regardless of any measure of the issue's "objective" importance.

But beyond sheer amount of coverage there is another aspect of news gatekeeping—that of emphasis and color. In a content analysis of three popular magazines from 1959 through 1974, Fisher et al. (1981) found women to be held responsible for male heart disease. "They are admonished to take actions that will either prevent or ameliorate male heart disease" (p. 255). Freimuth et al. (1984) have neatly laid out the "established chain of scientific information flow through professional communicators and science writers" (p. 62), and report content analyses of cancer articles from the top 50 U.S. newspapers in 1977 and 1980. *Prevention* of cancer was mentioned in only 6% of news stories in 1980 and 4% in 1977. A similarly small proportion mentioned detection (3% and 2%, respectively) or warning signs (6%, 2%). News stories tended to emphasize "dying rather than coping" (p. 70); human interest stories constituted only 7% each year. The authors noted their findings support a notion of cancer news coverage as "fragmented and ephemeral, which . . . may seriously affect the public's understanding of the disease" (p. 72).

Health professionals tend to blame the media for inaccurate reporting, and media professionals tend to return the blame. Williams (1975) noted that popular press publications are often the primary source of medical information for individuals. Finding this trend "dangerous." he called for restrictions via medical self-regulation and official gatekeeping. Responding to this, newspaper editor Shaun McIlraith (1975) admitted that a "God-like" image of the physician has been cultivated by the media, but in rebuttal stated that there has not been much effort by medicine to correct this view.

News coverage may affect the attitudes an individual holds toward health professionals and institutions. A phone survey of Ohio adults found a direct relationship between perceived positive news coverage of health care and positive perceptions of health care—but less so for one's own health care than for health care in society at large (Culbertson & Stempel, 1985).

AN OVERVIEW OF ENTERTAINMENT MEDIA INFLUENCE
(LINKS 1 AND 2)

That media content intended solely for entertainment purposes may result in unintended cognitive, affective, and behavioral impacts is not under debate. What is less certain is how these impacts occur, and what generates the individual differences. As noted earlier, social learning theory has received wide support in studies on media effects. A cognitive variation on this theory, Gerbner's (1980) cultivation theory, states that repeated exposure to consistent images of a TV world will create beliefs and expectations about the real world. Heavy TV viewers, for example, are found to be more fearful of what they perceive to be a crime-ridden real world. Clearly, such possibilities have important implications for how the individual *learns* about health and health professionals, what *attitudes* she or he holds about health, and how she or he *behaves* in a real-world health situation. Few studies have been able to assess impacts directly, so we inferentially make cautious assessments from studies of the health messages themselves.

Content analyses have given us baseline information on what effects may be occurring, having been applied to such diverse entertainment media as TV soap operas (Greenberg, Neuendorf, Buerkel-Rothfuss, & Henderson, 1982) and newspaper comic strips (Sofalvi & Drolet, 1986). A 1963 analysis of prime-time TV programming found 35 hours per week devoted to science, with the overwhelming majority (76%) devoted to medicine and psychology (61% of this content was fiction). "The mass media view of science is predominantly one concerned with the ills and aches, the mending and fixing of man's sick body and mind" (Sherburne, 1963, pp. 303–304).

Over the years, the world of television has continued to be one in which a vastly disproportionate number of physicians practice, yet, outside of designated medical programs, few people suffer pain or seek medical help. In spite of television entertainment's violent mayhem of chasing and shooting, its world is sanitized of blood and pain, and few require medical attention. When physicians practice, long-term aspects of treatment of chronic conditions are downplayed in favor of short-term biomedical treatment (Turow, 1985). Only 2% of all characters have been portrayed as physically handicapped, and about 7% of all major characters have had injuries or illnesses requiring attention (Gerbner, Morgan & Signorielli, 1982). However, in the world of entertainment TV there is considerable talk about health; two studies spanning a decade have found health to be the most prominent topic of conversation on TV soap operas (Greenberg et al., 1982; Katzman, 1972).

The health content of soap operas has been scrutinized in several studies, and appropriately so—soap fans tend to watch specifically so that they may see others dealing with social and personal problems, many of them health related. Soaps also have a long history of social scientific investigation, dating back to content analyses and listener surveys in the 1940s. James Thurber (1948, cited in Cassata, Skill, & Boadu, 1983) identified illness as a major theme in radio soaps, with "temporary blindness, amnesia, and paralysis of the legs" (p. 48) the top three adult afflictions. Soap children were stricken with "pneumonia and strange fevers, automobile accidents, and death through mysterious illnesses," whereas in real life cancer and infantile paralysis were the scourge. A New York psychiatrist accused radio soaps of causing increased blood pressure, tremors, and vertigo in their listeners (p. 50).

Greenberg et al. (1982) found 16% of all problems discussed on a sample of 1977 soaps to be medical in nature (down from 24% in 1970); the primary origin of these problems shifted over time as well, with less physical disability and more mental illness in 1977, and new "sex-related" problems occurring only in 1977. Thirteen percent of all conversations occurred in hospitals and 21% of all conversations dealt with health. The authors did not, however, find an agenda-setting function as to problems in a survey of female soap viewers.

A content analysis of *Soap Opera Digest* summaries of daytime soaps for all of 1977 (Cassata et al., 1983) identified 191 instances of health-related conditions for the 341 characters in 13 soaps; 22.5% of these terminated in the character's death. Forty-one percent of health problems were accidental/violent. These included car accidents, the second leading cause of death on soaps (compared to fourth in real life—5.3 annual deaths per 100 characters vs. 0.022 per 100 persons in real life; p. 61), homicides (2.9 per 100 on soaps vs. 0.009 per 100 in real life) and suicides (0.88 per 100 on soaps vs. 0.013 per 100 in real life). Twenty-one percent of health occurrences were diseases of the organs (largely cardiovascular, thereby accurately presenting heart disease as a top health threat). The remaining 32% were distributed over the categories of psychiatric disorders, pregnancy-related conditions, and symptomatic illnesses (p. 55). Most pregnancies were "unhappy." No soap characters died of cancer, America's number 2 real life killer. Most health problems occurred to those in the 22- to 45-age range. Women were less mentally stable and died at a greater rate from cardiovascular disease.

What effect do these images of health have on receivers? Fewer studies have made this more difficult assessment. Sherburne (1963) reported on a 1958 survey asking 541 TV viewers to name the programs that were sources of their science information.

> "Medic," the prime time drama series about doctors, was regarded by 30.5% as their chief source of science news. "Disneyland" attracted 10.0%, followed by "Medical Horizons," a medical documentary with 9.2%. And astonishingly enough, 4.8% listed the General Electric commercials, and 3.3% a daytime soap opera "Dr. Hudson's Secret Journal." (pp. 300–301)

A study by General Mills (1979, cited in Gerbner et al., 1982) asked respondents to select two or three main personal sources of information from a list of 16 potential sources (including doctors and dentists, families, television programs, and friends). Although "doctors and dentists" was the most-cited source (45%), second place fell to "television programs" (31%). More telling, those who chose TV programs as a major source were found to be significantly more complacent about health, more likely to hold "old" health values, less likely to exercise, and more poorly informed about health.

Clearly, some receivers tend to treat fictional health presentations as real. Anecdotal evidence supports this contention. Davidson (1973) reported a number of hypochondriacal—and life-saving—examples of information gleaned from TV shows by viewers. In one case, an 11-year-old boy saved his asthmatic brother's life with a rough version of the CPR he had seen on "Marcus Welby, M.D." Self-diagnosis by patients in nursing homes is not uncommon.

If we may safely assume that entertainment images of health—particularly those on television—create belief systems for receivers, then there may also be generational effects at work. Sandman (1976) noted, "One generation of patients and doctors grew up with Ben Casey and Dr. Kildare. Another generation is growing up with Marcus Welby and Joe Gannon" (p. 381). Figure 7.2 presents a timeline from 1951 through mid-1988 showing the number of hours per week devoted to health-based programs on prime-time network television. This presentation does *not* include (a) syndicated programs (e.g., "Dr. Simon Locke"), (b) daytime soap operas (e.g., "The Doctors," "General Hospital"), and (c) other media content.[3] We see essentially two eras of TV health shows—the 1960's world of ultra-serious medical drama with God-like physicians in neophyte-and-mentor contexts (e.g., "Ben Casey" and his Dr. Zorba, "Dr. Kildare" and his Dr. Gillespie; Newcomb, 1974), and the 1970's–1980's dual-image world of serious-but-very-human health professionals (e.g., "St. Elsewhere") and funny-but-empathic medicine (e.g., "M*A*S*H"). There were essentially no medical comedies prior to "M*A*S*H," but many have followed (and most have since fallen by the wayside).

CONTENT AREAS

Nutrition and Body Image

Identifying guidelines for good nutrition, Kaufman (1980) proceeded to show how TV violates them all. In a 1977 content analysis of the top 10 prime-time programs, she found repeated and consistent violations of the eight tenets, including: "restrict consumption of sugar" (19% of the total TV diet was desserts and sweets); "do not eat between meals"

---

[3]Documentation for such media content is generally unavailable, and the average exposure rate to TV has long exceeded exposure to other media by several-fold.

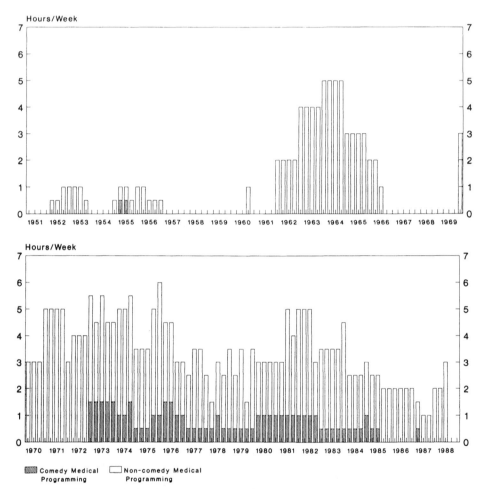

FIG. 7.2. Medical prime-time network television programming, 1951–
1988 (Sources: Brooks & Marsh, 1988; Terrace, 1976).

(in fewer than 20% of all eating instances did characters actually eat
a meal); and "give full attention to what you eat; do not eat 'on the go' "
(TV characters usually ate while primarily engaged in some other
behavior). Characters never ate explicitly to satisfy hunger—rather,
they ate to "fulfill social and psychological needs" (p. 43). At the same
time, only 12% were found to be overweight.

Gerbner et al. (Gerbner, Gross, Morgan, & Signorielli, 1981a;
Gerbner et al., 1982) have found similar trends in obesity and in
snacking on prime-time TV. "Grabbing a snack (39 percent of all
eating–drinking episodes) is virtually as frequent as breakfast, lunch,
and dinner combined (42 percent). In weekend-daytime children's pro-

grams, snacks go up to 45 percent, and regular meals decline to 24 percent, with 'other meals' making up the rest. The snack is fruit in only 4% or 5% of these episodes" (Gerbner et al., 1982, p. 296). Yet, in the same analyses of 1979 programming, only 6% of males and 2% of females—and none of them leading characters—were obese.

It must be noted that television nutrition has changed since the times of these studies. Bill Cosby's Dr. Huxtable fights the constant battle of the bulge, and is sometimes shamed into practicing good nutrition by his offspring. And the young women stars of "The Facts of Life" were portrayed as elegant and attractive in spite of their not-insubstantial girth.

Indeed, young females are most likely to be affected by body-image messages. Freedman (1984) noted the tendency for adolescent females to be caught-up in the development of their own narcissistic self-image, and therefore to be in need of collecting images. She cited studies showing the effect of magazine ads and TV spots on teenage images of beauty. "The ideal female physique that is currently considered attractive is further from the physiological norm than the male physique" (p. 35), she concluded.

That this current ideal type is media created is in little doubt. Swartz (1987) reasonably noted that anorexia is limited to Western females, clearly a response to sociocultural factors, and decried the present lack of definitive studies showing a clear link between media exposure and anorexic behavior. Again, the issue is clouded by the lack of specification of *mechanisms* by which the individual learns and has attitude. Even effects of rational pro-health appeals are not clear cut. Some physicians have even encountered a type of "negative learning," as when "vomiting as a weight control technique was learned by some . . . patients through . . . public education" aimed at eliminating the bulemic behavior (p. 616).

Mental Illness

Chief among the health-stigmatized population in our society in general and on television in particular are the mentally ill. Early attention was given to media treatments of the mentally ill by Gerbner (1959, 1961; Gerbner & Tannenbaum, 1960). Investigating mental health coverage by popular print media, films, and TV from 1900 through 1959, he concluded that mental health information follows the "economic trends of the nation. Popular interest in (or exposure to) articles on mental illness, psychiatry and psychology appears to rise in war and prosperity and fall during depression or recession" (Gerbner, 1961, p. 92).

He also examined TV network censorship files during the 1950s (Gerbner, 1959), finding an increase in the treatment of mental illness in feature films cleared for broadcast, as well as an increase in censorial cuts. The words most often deleted, in descending order, were: "Crazy," "idiot," "moron," "nuts," "screwy," "imbecile," "psychiatry," "feebleminded," "lunatic," "looney," and "half-wit" (p. 301). The censorship of mental illness content in films and TV changed slowly from a taboo against merely mentioning the "unpleasantness" of insanity to a real sensitivity, avoiding crude descriptors of the mentally ill (Gerbner & Tannenbaum, 1960). In the list just given, we see mostly the latter, but a vestige of the former as well, in the prohibition of the term *psychiatry*.

Fruth and Padderud (1985) content analyzed 70 episodes of 14 daytime soaps, and found 7 containing featured portrayals of mentally ill individuals, with 4 others presenting information about mental illness indirectly through conversation by other characters. Of all program time, 11.4% was devoted to portrayals or discussions of mental illness (p. 386). All mentally ill were White and virtually all were aged 22-45. Six of eight were women. These portrayals seem likely to perpetuate stigmatization, in that they also tended to show the mentally ill as criminal, dangerous, "different" in appearance, and not involved in psychiatric therapy.

The Cassata et al. (1983) work on soap operas cited earlier found the preponderance of TV characters with psychiatric disorders to be female, and most professionals with such a disorder were themselves health professionals. Psychiatric disorders were the number one specific health-related problem in the soap-opera world of 1977.

In a nonscientific Media Watch, Wahl and Roth (1982) monitored prime-time programming on five channels in Washington, D.C., during 1981. Of the 385 program episodes viewed, 29% had some mental health content; 19% had minor reference to mental illness and 9% contained mentally ill characters. The mentally ill tended to be identified "only by their mental illness" (p. 604), that is, their family roles, marital stati, and occupations were routinely left unspecified. They tended to be described by the volunteer viewers as "active," "confused," and "aggressive."

Distilling 240 different mental health-related statements from public opinions (200 interviews), mental health profession publications, media news and entertainment content, Nunnally (1957) presented these as Likert-type items to 349 respondents. In this most comprehensive of studies on media and perceptions of the mentally ill, cluster analysis revealed 10 clusters, which then served as the basis for a 1954 content analysis of 50 newspapers, 91 magazines, 1 TV station's weekly offerings, and a week's content of 4 radio stations. The 10 cluster categories of perceptions were also presented for response to a general population sample and a sample of 40 "experts." The opinions of the experts and the general public did not differ substantially, but the media images did diverge on several clusters. In comparison to attitudes of experts and the general public, media content displayed a greater tendency to portray the mentally ill as looking and acting "different," and to characterize mental illness as organically based, avoidable if one does not succumb to "morbid thoughts," and helped by guidance and support from a "strong" person in the environment. Further analyses of these data found mental health content in entertainment TV to be concentrated in crime drama and soap operas. Media portrayals of therapists, especially psychiatrists, evoked descriptors such as "clean," "good," and "intelligent" (Taylor, 1957, p. 201).

Work specifically examining how *news* information has impacted on receivers has concentrated on coverage of the criminally insane and of suicides.[4] A survey of 413 Albany respondents found clear differences between the aggregate perception of "mental patients" and "criminally insane patients" (Steadman & Cocozza, 1977–1978). Forty-two percent were able to name a newsworthy person who they thought was "criminally insane"—but most were famous murderers or assassins who had not been legally classified in that manner.

Imitative suicide is not a new concern. Johann Wolfgang Goethe's *The Sorrows of Werther,* written in 1774, was the source of imitative suicides for decades to follow (Gabe, 1987, p. 19-A). This story of a jilted lover's suicide gave rise to the term *Werther effect.* Present-day investigations of the Werther effect (Phillips, 1974, 1977, 1979) have found suicides and single-car automobile fatalities (as potential "disguised" suicides) to increase significantly after a suicide has been publicized in newspaper stories.

Substance Use and Abuse

As implied earlier, probably the most "abused" substance on TV is food, but there are even more hazardous images abounding. The depiction of use and abuse, and even the promotion, of hazardous substances such as tobacco products, alcoholic beverages, and illicit drugs are common in media. Smoking of tobacco products is on the wane both in real life and in the media, and was never extremely prevalent on TV (Greenberg, Fernandez-Collado, Graef, Korzenny, & Atkin, 1980). Alcohol consumption has been another matter.

Gerbner and his colleagues (1982) found over one third of all prime-time TV characters were alcohol users, but only 1% were abusers (alcoholics and/or drinking to excess); Greenberg, Fernandez-Collado et al. (1980) found only 6% shown using alcohol. A 1975 study determined the imbibing rate in soap operas to be 8.5 alcoholic beverages per hour

---

[4]See Matas, el-Guebaly, Peterkin, Green, and Harper (1985) for a bibliography on other aspects of mental illness and factual media.

versus 7.4 soft drinks per hour (Lowery, 1980). Similarly, 62% of the acts of beverage drinking identified in a 1977 study of situation comedies and dramas involved alcohol (Breed & DeFoe, 1981). A 1976–1978 study found an average of over two acts of consumption per hour, with the most frequent drinking occurring on crime dramas and sitcoms (Greenberg, Fernandez-Collado et al., 1980).

The studies found typical TV drinkers to be male, mature adults, and of all socioeconomic backgrounds. In a surprising example of how the context of drinking may be important, one analysis found that drinking occurred during or just before work in 25% of cases. Heavy drinking was excused or rationalized in 39% of the sitcom drinking cases; the usual mechanism was humor (Breed & DeFoe, 1981).

Drinking is often depicted as a means of dealing with stress or as a way to relax in conversation with friends (Lowry, 1981). As one 16-year-old respondent evaluated a "Cheers" bar scene, "It was useful; it made them feel better and they made friends" (Neuendorf, 1985, p. 76). This framing of alcohol in a positive light is not limited to TV—a study of best selling novels from 1900 to 1904 and 1946 to 1950 found two thirds of the frequent drinking instances to be projecting an image of alcohol as "supportive and good," most shown as supporting social relationships (Pfautz, 1962). But at the same time that users are portrayed positively, "abusers" (alcoholics) are assigned very negative images in all media (Cook & Lewington, 1979).

The promotion of liquor via alcohol advertising also helps build a context of support for consumption. Although links of exposure to alcohol advertising to immediate drinking behavior have not been established, those heavily exposed tend to think more positively of typical drinkers, and youngsters are more likely to drink to excess (Atkin, Neuendorf, & McDermott, 1983; Neuendorf, 1987).

Illicit drug use is far less sanctioned—the few studies assessing its prevalence in entertainment TV have found it to be negligible (Greenberg, Fernandez-Collado et al., 1980; McEwen & Hanneman, 1974). Recent films have dealt more explicitly with drugs' growing presence in society (e.g., *The River's Edge*), and of course will be appearing on pay cable TV. Concern has been evidenced over rock music lyrics that promote drug abuse. In addition, the spectre of an American "drugged-out" on *legal*, over-the-counter drugs has also been raised by those concerned with a plethora of over-the-counter drug ads promising health and happiness (see, for example, Ostman, 1976).

Aging

The graying of America has resulted in a lagged graying of the entertainment media. From "The Golden Girls" to "Cocoon," older positive images are turning around the trends of many years, during which time the elderly were very infrequently portrayed, and when they were, they tended to be sickly or feeble minded, or else bad tempered ("crotchety") and the butt of humor (Aronoff, 1974; Gantz, Gartenberg, & Rainbow, 1980; Greenberg, Korzenny, & Atkin, 1980).

One study of elderly TV viewers found that the more they perceived the elderly on TV as portrayed as "hindrances" to society (i.e., feeble minded, physically ill, a burden to society), the lower was their own self-concept (Korzenny & Neuendorf, 1980). More and more, however, media are presenting the aged with positive images to emulate, rather than reminders only of the negative aspects of aging.

Sexual Behaviors

Not too many years ago, those looking at sexual behaviors in the media took a *moral* approach—was the sex act portrayed in the context of a love relationship, and so on. (See Neuendorf, 1982, for a review of this literature.) Today, sexual behaviors, in and out of the media, are *health-related* behaviors. First, concern with unwanted pregnancy and genital herpes, then AIDS, have shifted the emphases of criticism and examination.

Those media institutions that are trying to depict sexual activity as responsible and "safe" have had a long way to go. For many years, entertainment television has depicted a world of frequent sex (implied clearly about once per hour) and frequent talk about sex (another once per hour) (e.g., Greenberg, Abelman, & Neuendorf, 1981; Greenberg, Graef, Fernandez-Collado, Korzenny, & Atkin, 1980). Birth control was never mentioned. Fictional media sex was presented as heterosexual, romantic, having no negative consequences, and something to be done with someone to whom you are not married (sex between unmarrieds typically outnumbers sex between marrieds at a ratio of 3:1). Fictional media sex has looked so good, it could have deleterious comparative effects on young people's satisfaction with their own sex life (Baran, 1976a, 1976b).[5]

Today, one cannot escape a barrage of press stories about herpes and AIDS (Feldman & Johnson, 1986; Mirotznik & Mosellie, 1986). Entertainment media, however, preserve an escapist world where sexual partners still worry little about contracting disease or creating new life. Planned Parenthood has lambasted entertainment TV in its release of a content analysis it commissioned. "There's very little talk of birth control . . . [*Even*] [c]ontraceptive ads are not on because of network decision makers who think contraception is a woman's problem" (Lubrano, 1988, pp. 5-B, 10-B). Using a broader definition of sex than that usually employed, the Planned Parenthood study identified

---

[5]Thus creating a market for the "Dr. Ruth" show.

an average of 27 sex behaviors per hour of prime time TV, with only a tiny proportion presented in a context of consequences and responsibility.

Health Professional Roles

While working for the Michigan State Police during the mid-1970s I was privy to many examples of the clear effects of occupational roles learned from television. Citizens would insist that the officers could do very specialized tasks—and do them immediately—because they had "seen it on television."[6] Health professionals have complained of—and gloried in—the same type of halo effect. Cultivation theory would predict that repeated exposure to fictional images will foster what one might term a *Marcus Welby Syndrome,* an unusually strong tendency to believe that physicians are all-powerful and all-good.

This syndrome includes the unrealistic belief that doctors can spend unlimited time with each patient. Doctors and nurses on entertainment television occur at a rate of almost five times their real-life proportions. Greenberg et al. (1982) found 37% of all males with identifiable jobs on soaps to be doctors; 21% of all females with identifiable jobs were nurses—obviously, a huge disparity from real life. The typical TV viewer sees approximately 12 physicians and 6 nurses each week on prime-time TV (Gerbner et al., 1982, p. 293), hopefully more than she or he sees in real life.

Portrayals of TV health professionals are just as unrealistic as their numbers. Warner (1979, cited in Gerbner et al., 1982) found that 61% of TV doctors' duties were performed on house calls or in the field.

> The television physician ... thrives on private relationships with patients, and wields absolute authority over auxiliary medical personnel, but is rarely shown at home or with a spouse or family of his own. Television doctors give advice and orders twice as frequently to female patients or to patients' wives as to male patients or to patients' husbands. (p. 294)

Nurses, too, have been assigned a series of images over the years, from positive and supportive in the 1950s, to nondescript, background roles in the 1960s, to continued background contributions in the dramas of the 1970s and the various aborted attempts at medical humor (noted exception: "M*A*S*H"; Kalisch, Kalisch, & Scobey, 1983).

Table 7.1 shows the number of health professionals appearing as

---

[6]The police officers themselves were sometimes affected by police drama they had seen on TV, a potential source of self-aggrandizing among physicians.

TABLE 7.1
Health Professionals on Entertainment Prime-Time Network TV, 1951–1988

Year	Physicians (F/Min)		Nurses (M/Min)		Other (F/Min)	
1951	0		0		0	
1952	3	(1/0)	1		1	
1953	3	(1/0)	1		0	
1954	1		0		0	
1955	4		1		1	
1956	3		0		3	
1957	0		0		2	
1958	1		0		2	
1959	3		1		1	
1960	5		1		1	
1961	9	(1/0)	3		1	
1962	12	(1/0)	6		3	
1963	11	(1/0)	4		4	
1964	15	(1/0)	4		5	
1965	15	(1/0)	4		1	
1966	9	(1/0)	2		1	
1967	2		0		1	
1968	2		3	(0/1)	1	
1969	10	(1/0)	6	(0/2)	0	
1970	16	(2/1)	6	(0/2)	1	
1971	16	(2/1)	6	(0/2)	3	
1972	22	(2/1)	15	(0/2)	4	
1973	22	(2/1)	15	(0/2)	4	
1974	21	(2/1)	15	(0/2)	6	(1/0)
1975	22	(2/0)	17	(0/2)	5	
1976	27	(2/0)	22	(0/2)	7	(0/1)
1977	23	(2/0)	20	(0/1)	6	(0/1)
1978	17	(2/0)	17	(1/2)	5	(0/1)
1979	21	(1/1)	19	(0/1)	7	(2/1)
1980	14		13	(0/1)	4	(1/1)
1981	16		17	(0/1)	4	(1/1)
1982	32	(3/1)	19	(0/1)	6	(2/1)
1983	43	(6/2)	17	(0/1)	5	(1/1)
1984	27	(4/3)	11		2	(1/0)
1985	25	(4/3)	9		7	(1/1)
1986	27	(4/2)	8	(0/1)	2	
1987	19	(6/2)	4		5	(1/0)
1988 (Jan.–June)	23	(8/3)	4		2	

Note: Unbracketed numbers represent the total number of regular characters across all network prime-time programs who appeared as physicians, nurses, or other health professionals (e.g., medical technologists, psychologists, coroners) during a given year. The first number inside each pair of parentheses is the number of females in that total, and the second number is the number of minority individuals in that total. When no parentheses are given, it indicates that no minorities or individuals of nontraditional gender (i.e., female physicians and other health professionals, male nurses) for that job appeared as regular characters that year.
Source: Brooks & Marsh, 1988.

regular characters in prime-time network TV programming during the period 1951–mid-1988 (This includes *all* programming, not just those programs categorized for Fig. 7.2 as "health programs"). We see a population of physicians, nurses, and "other" health professionals that has generally been growing through the years.

Extreme gender stereotyping seems prevalent in health professional portrayals (Kalisch & Kalisch, 1984; McLaughlin, 1975). Doctors (males) are powerful, brave, and compassionate. Nurses (females) are subservient, extraneous, and aloof. Table 7.1 shows the dearth of cross-gender doctor and nurse models on TV, with some improvement in recent years. This dearth can have serious effects—Beuf's (1974) classic interviews with little girls who had to grow up to be "nothing," or would like to be doctors if only they were boys, remind us that sheer lack of models can be devastating. And it is clear that exposure to a single mass media example of a counter-stereotype can change attitudes about appropriate occupations for genders (see Busby, 1975, for an excellent, still timely review).

Turow (1985) noted that hospital and health-care *executives,* as well as those on the front lines, are given images by news and entertainment. He contended these images are largely negative, showing executives as "obstructions" to good medicine, and worried that this makes it "easier for policymakers to act negatively toward them in real life" (p. 97).

Therapeutic TV

Is there no good in entertainment media, and TV in particular? Are there no accurate, healthful, or helpful images? Just as 20 years of concentration on violent behaviors gave way to a grudging acknowledgment of the occurrence of *pro*-social learning, some health professionals have seemingly given in completely to the box. Television is being used as *treatment* in mental health and recuperative situations.

Early work by Bandura (1971) and others established television's capability to reduce fear and phobic responses through the display of models.[7] More recently, some researchers have used TV as a socializing agent for those in institutions (Falk-Kessler & Froschauer, 1978; Kilguss, 1974, 1977; Rubinstein & Sprafkin, 1982). Although some health professionals complain bitterly about the triviality of soap operas, others are using them in innovative projective therapy.

Others have developed video for closed-circuit hospital viewing (Dries & Ratazak, 1985), and video for children as a source of informa-

---

[7]For example, children viewing others playing safely with dogs were better able to overcome their own fear of dogs; similar findings have been found with regard to children's fear of dentists.

tion about other children who are hospitalized or handicapped (Graham, 1985; Guttentag, Albritton, & Kettner, 1981).[8] And, even the role of mediated humor as a healthful stimulant is just beginning to be explored (Mannell & McMahon, 1982).[9]

Work at the National Asthma Center has developed a technique called *self-modeling*:

> in which a child views himself over a TV monitor performing an act necessary to his well-being. Unfortunately, a large amount of modeling comes to the child in an unplanned fashion through commercial television where, in the US at least, violence and the use of food products are modeled, which probably contribute deleteriously to the child's health and well-being. (Burns, 1979, p. 9)

In this quote, Burns has both indicted the medium of television *and* redeemed it, showing its therapeutic potential and the commonly detrimental actuality.

FEEDBACK TO MEDIA FROM HEALTH PROFESSIONALS

Links 5 and 6 in the model shown in Fig. 7.1 recognize the importance of feedback from the health profession to media outlets. This feedback occurs in both formalized and nonformalized ways. Formalized feedback mechanisms include the AMA's Physicians Advisory Committee on Television, Radio and Motion Pictures (founded in 1955; Cobb, 1966) and the American Academy of Family Physicians' Public Relations Committee (both of which reviewed all "Marcus Welby" scripts; Real, 1977). Efforts by the American Nursing Association to provide input for the 1960's program "The Nurses" were rebuffed by the producers.

Nonformalized feedback can take interesting forms, from grassroots mobilization efforts (as proposed by, e.g., Friemuth et al., 1984; Sandman, 1976; Whelan, 1987) to the publication of sometimes scathing attacks by medical professionals in popular media (e.g., Goldberg, 1977; Halberstam, 1972; Rennie, 1973). Unfortunately, many such critiques are ineffectual, in that they flippantly dismiss the medically uninformed, with a figurative wave of the hand. For example, when "forced" to watch a week of TV and comment on it (he had to *rent* a set), one physician wrote he was so taxed by the ordeal, "I ask[ed] my daughter

---

[8]It should be noted that Guttentag et al.'s development of "alternative" educational video content resulted from their observational finding that hospitalized children's broadcast TV viewing is "indiscriminate and excessive" (p. 672).

[9]"Take two aspirin and three Marx Brothers, and call me in the morning" might be in the offing.

to fan me with a sterile hat while . . . I [had] another Schlitz" (Rennie, 1973, p. 23).

FUTURE TRENDS

Cable television, with its "something for everyone" grab bag of offer-ings, has at the same time made health information more accessible and more remote (by making it specialized). The Lifetime network, with its stated objective of providing "women's programming," has tightened the connection between health professionals and viewers. It offers a full day of health news and documentary content each Sunday, and several programs daily. The eighth most widespread basic service cable network as of May, 1987, it was available to over 32 million households via 3,310 cable systems and enjoyed a 19% increase in penetration over the previous 12 months (*Broadcasting/Cablecasting Yearbook*, 1988, p. D-364). Lifetime's Sunday smorgasbord of health includes such specialized factual programming as "Cardiology Update," "Orthopaedic Surgery Update," and "Age and Hypertension." A cursory perusal of this programming makes it clear that the intended audience includes health professionals as well as the general public; performers do not mince medical terminology.

More critical attention is also being paid to health images in enter-tainment content, especially in that most powerful of all media, televi-sion/cable. Health professionals have begun to put mass media channels high on their hit list of motivators that keep Americans in "unhealthy lifestyles" (Townes, 1984). Popular literature has gotten into the con-tent analysis act with nonscientific ratings of "healthy" and "un-healthy" TV. Author Michele Salcedo declared war on "cookie-junkie" "Webster," the nicotine, caffeine, and no-seat-belts of "Hill Street Blues," and the bar-hopping of "Miami Vice." The "all-around heroine" of the 1986 "rating" was Mary Beth Lacey of "Cagney and Lacey," who exercises, does not drink or smoke, and deals with stress in a positive fashion ("Keeping TV healthy," 1986, p. 22).

The popularity of Jane Fonda's workout video and of aerobics TV programs tells us that exercise is "in"—and visual media have been essential in imparting information about the obvious physical benefits of exercise. The benefits of other healthful activities are not always so observable, and so do not fit the relevant characteristics of today's fast-paced visual media. That is, one cannot *see* the results of a lifetime of nonsmoking in a 60-minute episode of "Heartbeat."

As media become more user driven, expanded formats will be possi-ble: A rented educational video on prevention of heart attacks can be viewed over and over; the wide selection of informative programs available on Lifetime may be videotaped for later use by a VCR owner. But with the good comes the bad: Cable TV has also brought back the infallible "Ben Casey"; home video gives complete gatekeeping power to the receiver to watch such unrealistic images as those in "Reefer Madness," "One Flew Over the Cuckoo's Nest," "Harvey," "The Dark Past," and "Dark Victory"—repeatedly.

ACKNOWLEDGMENT

Special thanks go to James Brentar for his invaluable assistance in the compilation of information for this chapter.

REFERENCES

Aronoff, C. (1974). Old age in prime time. *Journal of Communication, 24*(4), 86–87.
Atkin, C. K., Neuendorf, K., & McDermott, S. (1983). The role of alcohol advertising in excessive and hazardous drinking. *Journal of Drug Education, 13*, 313–325.
Bandura, A. (1969). Social-learning theory of identificatory processes. In D. A. Goslin (Ed.), *Handbook of socialization theory and research* (pp. 213–262). Chicago: Rand McNally.
Bandura, A. (1971). *Social learning theory.* Morristown, NJ: General Learning Press.
Bandura, A., & Walters, R. H. (1963). *Social learning and personality development.* New York: Holt, Rinehart & Winston.
Baran, S. J. (1976a). How TV and film portrayals affect sexual satisfaction in college students. *Journalism Quarterly, 20*, 468–473.
Baran, S. J. (1976b). Sex on TV and adolescent self-image. *Journal of Broadcasting, 20*, 61–68.
Beuf, A. (1974). Doctor, lawyer, household drudge. *Journal of Communication, 24*(2), 142–145.
Breed, W., & DeFoe, J. R. (1981). The portrayal of the drinking process on prime-time television. *Journal of Communication, 31*(1), 58–67.
Broadcasting/Cablecasting Yearbook 1988. (1988). Washington, DC: Broadcast Publications Inc.
Brooks, T., & Marsh, E. (1988). *The complete directory to prime time network TV shows: 1946-present, fourth edition.* New York: Ballantine Books.
Burns, K. L. (1979). Social learning theory and behavioral health care. *Psychotherapy and Psychosomatics, 32*, 6–15.
Busby, L. J. (1975). Sex-role research on the mass media. *Journal of Communication, 25*(4), 107–131.
Cassata, M., Skill, T., & Boadu, S. O. (1983). Life and death in the daytime television serial: A content analysis. In M. Cassata & T. Skill (Eds.), *Life on daytime television: Tuning-in American serial drama* (pp. 47–69). Norwood, NJ: Ablex.
Cobb, D. M., Jr. (1966). Advice on medical accuracy in the entertainment media. *Western Medicine, 7*, 313–316.

Cook, J., & Lewington, M. (Eds.). (1979). *Images of alcoholism*. London: British Film Institute.

Culbertson, H. M., & Stempel, G. H. (1985). "Media malaise": Explaining personal optimism and societal pessimism about health care. *Journal of Communication, 35*(2), 180–190.

Davidson, M. (1973, July 21). Viewer, heal thyself! *TV Guide*, pp. 21–24.

Dries, L., & Ratazak, J. (1985). Who said TV is just for entertainment. *The Diabetes Educator, 10*(4), 28–29.

Falk-Kessler, J., & Froschauer, K. H. (1978). The soap opera: A dynamic group approach for psychiatric patients. *American Journal of Occupational Therapy, 32*, 317–319.

Feldman, D. A., & Johnson, T. M. (Eds.). (1986). *The social dimensions of AIDS: Method and theory*. New York: Praeger Publishers.

Fisher, J., Gandy, H., Jr., & Janus, N. Z. (1981). The role of popular media in defining sickness and health. In E. G. McAnany, J. Schnitman, & N. Janus (Eds.), *Communication and social structure: Critical studies in mass media research* (pp. 240–257). New York: Praeger.

Freedman, R. J. (1984). Reflections on beauty as it relates to health in adolescent females. *Women and Health, 9*, 29–45.

Freimuth, V. S., Greenberg, R. H., DeWitt, J., & Romano, R. M. (1984). Covering cancer: Newspapers and the public interest. *Journal of Communication, 34*(1), 62–73.

Fruth, L., & Padderud, A. (1985). Portrayals of mental illness in daytime television serials. *Journalism Quarterly, 62*, 384–387, 449.

Gabe, C. (1987, January 24). Set children straight on TV suicide. *The Cleveland Plain Dealer*, pp. 19-A, 21-A.

Gandy, O. H., Jr. (1981). The economics of image building: The information subsidy in health. In E. G. McAnany, J. Schnitman, & N. Janus (Eds.), *Communication and social structure: Critical studies in mass media research* (pp. 204–239). New York: Praeger.

Gantz, W., Gartenberg, H. M., Rainbow, C. K. (1980). Approaching invisibility: Portrayal of the elderly in magazine advertisements. *Journal of Communication, 30*(1), 56–60.

Gerbner, G. (1959). Mental illness on television: A study of censorship. *Journal of Broadcasting, 3*, 293–303.

Gerbner, G. (1961). Psychology, psychiatry, and mental illness in the mass media: A study of trends, 1900-1959. *Mental Hygiene, 45*, 89–93.

Gerbner, G. (1980). Dreams that hurt: Mental illness in the mass media. In R. C. Baron, I. D. Rutman, & B. Klaczynska (Eds.), *The community imperative* (pp. 19–23). Philadelphia: Horizon House Institute.

Gerbner, G., Gross, L., Morgan, M., & Signorielli, N. (1981a). Health and medicine on television. *The New England Journal of Medicine, 305*(15), 901–904.

Gerbner, G., Gross, L., Morgan, M., & Signorielli, N. (1981b). Scientists on the TV screen. *Society, 18*(4), 41–44.

Gerbner, G., Morgan, M., & Signorielli, N. (1982). Programing health portrayals: What viewers see, say, and do. In D. Pearl, L. Bouthilet, & J. Lazar (Eds.), *Television and behavior: Ten years of scientific progress and implications for the eighties, Vol. II, Technical reviews* (pp. 291–307). Rockville, MD: U.S. Department of Health & Human Services.

Gerbner, G., & Tannenbaum, P. H. (1960). Regulation of mental illness content in motion pictures and television. *Gazette, 6*, 365–385.

Goldberg, M. (1977, May 14). A doctor examines TV's health shows. *TV Guide*, pp. 4–8.

Graham, E. S. (1985). Some uses of television with hospitalized and handicapped children. *Progress in clinical and biological research, 163*, 347–350.

Greenberg, B. S., Abelman, R., & Neuendorf, K. (1981). Sex and the soap operas: After-noon delight. *Journal of Communication, 31*(3), 83–89.

Greenberg, B. S., Fernandez-Collado, C., Graef, D., Korzenny, F., & Atkin, C. K. (1980). Trends in use of alcohol and other substances on television. In B. S. Greenberg (Ed.), *Life on television: Content analyses of U.S. TV drama* (pp. 137–195). Norwood, NJ: Ablex.

Greenberg, B. S., Graef, D., Fernandez-Collado, C., Korzenny, F., & Atkin, C. K. (1980). Sexual intimacy on commercial television during prime time. In B. S. Greenberg (Ed.), Life on television: Content analyses of U.S. TV drama (pp. 129–136). Norwood, NJ: Ablex.

Greenberg, B. S., Korzenny, F., & Atkin, C. K. (1980). Trends in the portrayal of the elderly. In B. S. Greenberg (Ed.), *Life on television: Content analyses of U.S. TV drama* (pp. 23–34). Norwood, NJ: Ablex.

Greenberg, B. S., Neuendorf, K., Buerkel-Rothfuss, N., & Henderson, L. (1982). The soaps: What's on and who cares? *Journal of Broadcasting, 26,* 519–535.

Guttentag, D. N., Albritton, W. L., & Kettner, R. B. (1981). Daytime television viewing by hospitalized children. *Pediatrics, 68,* 672–676.

Halberstam, M. (1972, January 16). An M.D. reviews Dr. Welby of TV. *New York Times Magazine,* pp. 12–13, 30, 32, 34–35, 37.

Health care TV ads continue to grow at sizzling pace. (1986, August 4). *Television/Radio Age,* pp. 69–70, 121–123.

Kalisch, P. A., & Kalisch, B. J. (1984). Sex-role stereotyping of nurses and physicians on prime-time television: A dichotomy of occupational portrayals. *Sex Roles, 10*(7/8), 533–553.

Kalisch, P. A., Kalisch, B. J., & Scobey, M. (1983). *Images of nurses on television.* New York: Springer.

Kalish, D. (1987, August). The doctor is in. *Marketing and Media Decisions,* 8–9.

Katzman, N. (1972). Television soap operas: What's been going on anyway? *Public Opinion Quarterly, 36,* 200–212.

Kaufman, L. (1980). Prime-time nutrition. *Journal of Communication, 30*(3), 37–46.

Keeping TV healthy. (1986, September 15). *Television-Radio Age,* p. 22.

Kilguss, A. F. (1974). Using soap operas as a therapeutic tool. *Social Casework, 55,* 525–530.

Kilguss, A. F. (1977). Therapeutic use of a soap opera discussion group with psychiatric in-patients. *Clinical Social Work Journal, 5,* 58–65.

Korzenny, F., & Neuendorf, K. (1980). Television viewing and self-concept of the elderly. *Journal of Communication, 30*(1), 71–80.

Lowery, S. A. (1980). Soap and booze in the afternoon: An analysis of alcohol use in daytime serials. *Journal of Studies on Alcohol, 41,* 829–838.

Lowry, D. T. (1981). Alcohol consumption patterns and consequences on prime time network TV. *Journalism Quarterly, 58,* 3–8.

Lubrano, A. (1988, January 30). Preaching sex without sermon: TV accused of one-sided indoctrination. *The Cleveland Plain Dealer,* pp. 5-B, 10-B.

Mannell, R. C., & McMahon, L. (1982). Humor as play: Its relationship to psychological well-being during the course of a day. *Leisure Sciences, 5*(2), 143–155.

Manoff, R. K. (1986, April 21). Health claims? Less is best. *Advertising Age,* pp. 18, 22.

Matas, M., el-Guebaly, N., Peterkin, A., Green, M., & Harper, D. (1985). Mental illness and the media: An assessment of attitudes and communication. *Canadian Journal of Psychiatry, 30,* 12–17.

McEwen, W. J., & Hanneman, G. J. (1974). The depiction of drug use in television program-ming. *Journal of Drug Education, 4,* 281–293.

McIlraith, S. (1975, March 22). Comment 2. *The Medical Journal of Australia,* pp. 399–401.

McLaughlin, J. (1975). The doctor shows. *Journal of Communication, 25*(3), 182–184.

Mirotznik, J., & Mosellie, B. M. (1986). Genital herpes and the mass media. *Journal of Popular Culture, 20*(3), 1–12.

Neuendorf, K. A. (1982). *Sexual social learning via television: An experimental assessment of the possible impacts of "vidsex."* Unpublished doctoral dissertation, Department of Communication, Michigan State University, MI.

Neuendorf, K. A. (1985). Alcohol advertising and media portrayals. *The Journal of the Institute for Socioeconomic Policy, X*(2), 67–78.

Neuendorf, K. A. (1987). Alcohol advertising: Evidence from social science. *Media Information Australia, 43,* 15–20.

Neuendorf, K. A., & Pearlman, R. (1988). *Alcohol as good food: Adolescents' responses to liqueur ads.* Paper presented to the Advertising Division at the annual meeting of the Association for Journalism and Mass Communication, Portland, OR.

Newcomb, H. (1974) *TV: The most popular art.* Garden City, NY: Anchor Books.

Nunnally, J. (1957). The communication of mental health information: A comparison of the opinions of experts and the public with mass media presentations. *Behavioral Science, 2,* 222–230.

Ostman, R. E. (Ed.). (1976). *Communication research and drug education.* Beverly Hills, CA: Sage.

Pfautz, H. W. (1962). Image of alcohol in popular fiction: 1900–1904 and 1946–1950. *Quarterly Journal of Studies on Alcohol, 23*(1), 131–146.

Phillips, D. P. (1974). The influence of suggestion on suicide: Substantive and theoretical implications of the Werther effect. *American Sociological Review, 39,* 340–354.

Phillips, D. P. (1977). Motor vehicle fatalities increase just after publicized suicide stories. *Science, 196,* 1464–1465.

Phillips, D. P. (1979). Suicide, motor vehicle fatalities, and the mass media: Evidence toward a theory of suggestion. *American Journal of Sociology, 84,* 1150–1174.

Real, M. R. (1977). *Mass-mediated culture.* Englewood Cliffs, NJ: Prentice-Hall.

Rennie, D. (1973, January). What you can learn about health from TV. *Today's Health,* pp. 22–26.

Rubinstein, E. A., & Sprafkin, J. N. (1982). Television and persons in institutions. In D. Pearl, L. Bouthilet, & J. Lazar (Eds.), *Television and behavior: Ten years of scientific progress and implications for the eighties, Vol. II, Technical reviews* (pp. 322–330). Rockville, MD: U.S. Department of Health & Human Services.

Sandman, P. M. (1976). Medicine and mass communications: An agenda for physicians. *Annals of Internal Medicine, 85,* 378–393.

Sherburne, E. G., Jr. (1963). Science on television: A challenge to creativity. *Journalism Quarterly, 40,* 300–305.

Simpkins, J. D., & Brenner, D. J. (1984). Mass media communication and health. In B. Dervin & M. J. Voigt (Eds.), *Progress in communication sciences* (Vol. 5, pp. 275–297). Norwood, NJ: Ablex.

Sofalvi, A. J., & Drolet, J. C. (1986). Health-related content of selected Sunday comic strips. *Journal of School Health, 56*(5), 184–187.

Steadman, H. J., & Cocozza, J. J. (1977–1978). Selective reporting and the public's misconceptions of the criminally insane. *Public Opinion Quarterly, 41,* 523–533.

Swartz, L. (1987). Illness negotiation: The case of eating disorders. *Social Science and Medicine, 24*(7), 613–618.

Taylor, W. L. (1957). Gauging the mental health content of the mass media. *Journalism Quarterly, 34,* 191–201.

Terrace, V. (1976). *The complete encyclopedia of television programs 1947–1976.* South Brunswick: A. S. Barnes.

Townes, C. D. (1984). Wellness: The emerging concept and its components. *Individual Psychology Journal of Adlerian Theory, Research and Practice, 40*(4), 372–383.

Turow, J. (1985, November–December). Hospital and healthcare executives on TV: Image problems for the profession. *Hospital & Health Services Administration, 30,* 96–105.

Wahl, O. F., & Roth, R. (1982). Television images of mental illness: Results of a metropolitan Washington media watch. *Journal of Broadcasting, 26,* 599–605.

Whelan, E. M. (1987, November 1). Health hoax and a health scare. *Vital Speeches,* pp. 57–61.

Williams, F. (1982). *The communications revolution.* Beverly Hills, CA: Sage.

Williams, S. E. (1975, March 22). Medicine and the mass media. *The Medical Journal of Australia,* pp. 395–397.

8

Public Health Campaigns:
Individual Message Strategies and a Model

Lewis Donohew
University of Kentucky

Use of the mass media to persuade persons to engage in or avoid specific behaviors has been a subject of research for many years, but effective means of accomplishing this remain relatively elusive. Early experimental research dealt with such questions as the level of fear appeals in getting people to brush their teeth (Janis & Feshbach, 1953) and early survey research with the effectiveness of mass media in persuading individuals to vote for particular candidates (Berelson, Lazarsfeld, & McPhee, 1954; Lazarsfeld, Berelson, & Gaudet, 1948).

For a long time, research on persuasion was influenced by findings from these and similar studies that led to communication models that assumed a relatively high level of rationality on the part of the receivers (Festinger, 1964; Zajonc, 1968) and a largely ineffectual mass media in efforts to bring about behavior change (Klapper, 1960). This was reinforced by failure of various campaigns to produce desired results.

The history of public health campaigns in particular has been a story of expensive failures. Although reviews of recent research show some increased effectiveness in recent years (Flay, 1986; Flay, DiTecco, & Schlegel, 1980; Flay & Sobel, 1983), success stories continue to be relatively rare. Prominent among the reasons for failures is that expectations of direct media effects on behavior have been too ambitious. Another is that messages have failed to reach their target audiences. The principal question to be addressed here is: How do we get people to seriously attend to health information they need to have?

In this chapter, we describe evolving assumptions about the nature of human information processing that require a radical revision of the behavior-change expectations of the past and attention to the physiological as well as the cognitive properties of messages. From the perspective of the individual, the "rational" models of human behavior are giving way to more complex models of human beings as information processors, guided by both cognitive (Lazarus, 1982) and affective (Zajonc, 1980, 1984) forces.

We draw upon these models to propose a new approach to design of health campaigns involving the mass media. From a systems perspective, this approach continues to treat individuals as intrapersonal cybernetic systems, as in many previous studies by other investigators, but it updates the definition of the guiding mechanisms of those systems to take recent research on arousal, attention, and cognition into account and it considers the operation of these systems in a health environment.

The research findings in our field indicate that there are practical reasons for investigating the factors that affect the various aspects of message selection and processing, especially in terms of targeting audiences for specific kinds of persuasive messages, such as those aimed at drug abuse prevention. Unfortunately, most research addressed to the effectiveness of public health campaigns has paid little attention to the roles played by human information processing and individual differences in attracting and holding the attention of their target audiences (Donohew, Helm, Cook, & Shatzer, 1987).

In this chapter, we trace these connections in more detail and describe evolution of an affective–cognitive model of information exposure that has led to targeting and design of messages based on recent advances in these areas.

Neuendorf (chapter 7, this volume) wrote about the way messages ordinarily are prepared to be "palatable to one and all," and Brown and Einseidel (chapter 9) have written of ways they might be targeted to specific groups. In this chapter, it is assumed that multiple messages are designed with the expectation that some will appeal to one targeted group and some to another. Clearly, there is a limit on how many messages should be offered on a topic to avoid confusing those who attend to all of them and, practically, because there are limits on how many a campaign can afford to produce.

The reviews cited previously as well as others (Caplaces & Starr, 1973; Delaney, 1978; Rappaport, Labow, & Williams, 1975) indicate that little attention has been paid to evolving evidence about the nature of human information processing (Bargh, 1984, 1988; Cacioppo, Petty, & Tassinary, 1988; Donohew, Sypher, & Cook, 1988; Donohew, Sypher, & Higgins, 1988; Roloff, 1980), physiological arousal (Bryant & Zillmann, 1984; Christ, 1985; Christ & Biggers, 1984; Christ & Medoff,

1984; Finn, 1985a, 1985b; Zillmann, 1988a, 1988b; Zillmann & Bryant, 1985), or individual differences (Zuckerman, 1978, 1983, 1988) that offer opportunities for special targeting of messages and programs.

A principal benefit of such efforts can be more effective targeting of primary high-risk groups, the attraction of greater numbers of persons to call hotlines or otherwise become motivated to be involved in programs in which there are face-to-face interactions, and laying the groundwork for more effective persuasion to engage in healthful, prosocial activities.

Evidence of a general rethinking about information processing and decision-making capacities of human beings is emerging from more recent studies. From the perspective of the individual, the "rational" model of human behavior is giving way to more complex models of human beings as information processors, guided both by cognitive (Lazarus, 1982) and affective (Zajonc, 1980, 1984) forces.

The changing role of cognition and affect or arousal in communication was recently reviewed by a panel of nationally prominent psychologists and communication researchers (Donohew, Sypher, & Higgins, 1988). Their review reflects a more complex view of human beings as sometimes operating on subroutines of which they are only dimly aware (Bargh, 1988), such as those employed while driving home from work, and sometimes selecting communication stimuli such as television programs to help manage their moods (Zillmann, 1988a, 1988b). The level of arousal they need varies across individuals (Zuckerman, 1988) and affects the kinds of stimuli they will be likely to attend (Donohew, Finn, & Christ, 1988). It is apparent from existing research that these differences can significantly affect responses (Donohew, Palmgreen, & Duncan, 1980; Zuckerman, 1978, 1983).

This perspective is more consistent with what we know of humans as biological creatures, employing attention processes shaped by millions of years of evolution. For our primeval ancestors, a slight change in the coloration of a leaf or the presence of a subtle odor could lead to life-threatening or life-sustaining experiences, triggering arousal responses (Franklin, Donohew, Dhoundiyal, & Cook, 1988). To the present, we continue to respond to novelty with alertness and to familiarity with relaxation.

Research on sensation seeking has found that levels of need for arousal vary greatly across individuals (Zuckerman, 1978, 1983, 1988) and that high need for sensation is related to higher involvement with drugs. Zuckerman and others found that 74% of college undergraduates scoring high on his sensation-seeking scale (SSS) had used one or more drugs as opposed to 23% of those scoring low on the scale. Using a variety of personality measures, Segal and Singer (1976) found that the SSS provided the most discrimination between nonusers and various user groups. Use of specific drugs, such as amphetamines, marijuana, hashish, and LSD, correlates strongly with sensation seeking. Positive relationships were found between alcohol use and the disinhibition scale of the SSS in adolescents (Bates, Labouvier, & White, n.d.) and college students populations (Schwarz, Burkhart, & Green, 1978). Studies conducted with drug abusers found that medium and high sensation seekers had experimented with drugs at an earlier age than low sensation seeking abusers, and had more varied drug experience (Zuckerman, 1978).

Recent research by Donohew and associates (Donohew, 1988; Donohew, Helm, Cook, & Shatzer, 1987) on junior and senior high school students extends this relationship to youngsters in early and middle adolescence. The data offer strong support for employment of sensation seeking as an avenue for targeting prime at-risk groups and designing messages and programs to reach them. The studies consistently indicate highly significant differences in marijuana use between high and low sensation seekers at both the junior and senior high school levels. Among junior high school students, high sensation seekers clearly were the first to start using marijuana. Table 8.1 shows differences between high and low sensation seekers across a range of popular drugs at the junior and senior high school levels.

A further complication pointing to need for targeting is that persons with a high need for sensation tend to tolerate or even require stronger messages for attracting and holding their attention than persons with a lower need (Donohew, Finn, & Christ, 1988; Donohew et al., 1980).

Depending on the nature of a given stimulus message and how much it directly involves the subject, it may generate considerable excitement

TABLE 8.1
Sensation Seeking and Drug Use Among
Junior and Senior High School Students*

	Marijuana	Cocaine	Liquor	Beer	Uppers	Downers
Junior high LSS						
n = 658	6.2	.6	20.7	24.9	1.4	.5
Junior high HSS						
n = 565	24.7	3.4	58.3	58.3	14.9	11.2
Senior high LSS						
n = 450	13.0	1.8	28.5	38.0	2.0	1.6
Senior high HSS						
n = 420	38.3	6.6	67.1	70.5	14.8	6.6

*These figures represent percentage of students at the 7th- through 12th-grade levels who indicated use of particular drugs at least once during the last 30 days.

or it may be largely ignored as the subject moves on to something providing more stimulation.

The background for the revised model for health campaigns involving the mass media is drawn from three paradigms:

1. evolving theories of controlled and automatic information processing (see, for example, Bargh, 1984, 1988; Franklin et al., 1988; Langer, 1980; Roloff, 1980; Shiffrin & Schneider, 1977);
2. research on sensation seeking (Pearson, 1970, 1971; Zuckerman, 1978, 1983; Zuckerman, Kolin, Price, & Zoob, 1964);
3. an activation theory of information exposure (Donohew, Finn, & Christ, 1988; Donohew et al., 1980).

THEORETICAL BACKGROUND

Human beings are continuously involved in a search for stimulation, driven by pleasure centers of the midbrain (Olds & Fobes, 1981). It has been known for nearly a century that they find arousal in moderate amounts to be pleasurable (Wundt, 1874). This response to moderate arousal soon became connected with optimal behavior in an inverted U-curve (Yerkes & Dodson, 1908). At the lower end of this curve, arousal is too low to motivate performance. Beyond this and up to an optimal point, arousal has positive motivating values. After that point is passed, its value tends to be negative and inversely related to performance (Hebb, 1955). Berlyne (1971) hypothesized that the Wundt curve arises from the activation of both a pleasure system and an aversive system, with the pleasure system having a lower threshold of activation.

In summary, current arousal theories hold that behavioral efficiency increases as arousal increases to some optimal level, then falls off as the arousal level continues to increase (Cacioppo & Petty, 1983).

As previously described, need for arousal is fundamental to human behavior and serves an important function in the mechanisms guiding exposure to information. The more arousal potential a stimulus has, the more attention will be devoted to it (Martindale, 1981). Up to a point, increasing attention will be accompanied by increasing pleasure; beyond this point, increasing attention will be accompanied by increasing displeasure (Martindale, 1981).

It is generally agreed that attention, perception, comprehension, storage, and recall comprise the major psychological aspects of human information processing. In addition, research has demonstrated that the overall process is initiated not only by stimulus characteristics but also by the individual's level of physiological arousal (Cacioppo & Petty, 1983), a necessary condition upon which the human central nervous system depends for conscious, focused attention to any stimulus (Luria, 1973). Furthermore, it has long been known that arousal levels vary among individuals, and that this factor can account, at least in part, for selectivity in the attention process.

Information Processing

Recent research on information processing indicates that stimulus selection is accompanied by both cognitive and affective processes that range along a broad continuum, from controlled to automatic (Bargh, 1984; Langer, 1980). Under automatic processing, people's behavior is guided largely by processes of which they are not aware, but which they have overlearned in many previous repetitions (Schank & Abelson, 1977). For example, the process of driving one's car home, once underway, often is carried out automatically, allowing the driver to devote more time to other activities involving more novelty or greater effort, or to some other behaviors that tend to generate moderate and pleasurable arousal responses.

The interplay of controlled and automatic processing, the arousal response and stimulus properties, are what undergird stimulus selection. If something new or important appears while the homeward-bound driver is on automatic pilot, such as the flashing lights and siren of an emergency vehicle, he or she will shift attention to the new stimulus. This alert state usually will lead to an increase in controlled processing, as the driver concentrates on strategies to safely maneuver the car so that the emergency vehicle may pass. Once the threat of danger is dealt with, the response, as in driving, once again will become automatic. If the driver has experienced increased arousal in the process of coping with the traffic situation, he or she may change the radio dial from a rock station to a source of a more soothing sound without being aware of doing so. Attending to television, as another example, need not be for the controlled purpose of obtaining information, but for managing one's mood, which may be done more or less automatically. The individual who seems to "mindlessly" flip through the channels may be searching for the program which can meet his or her needs for arousal maintenance (Bryant & Zillmann, 1984; Zillmann, 1988a, 1988b; Zillmann & Bryant, 1985).

This switching back and forth between responses guided primarily by overlearned scripts and arousal and those guided in controlled processing by our cognitions is roughly analogous to the states described in the activation model in which individuals switch to consistency-seeking or variety-seeking states depending on their cognitive and activation responses to the environment.

Sensation Seeking

Although the activation model described earlier was designed to predict information exposure, it could be extended to include any source of stimulation, including drugs. One of its key elements is individual need for sensation, usually measured with a sensation-seeking scale (SSS) developed by Zuckerman (1978).

Variations in levels of need for physiological arousal form the basis for study of this psychological trait, referred to as sensation seeking, which has been investigated and measured since the 1960s (Pearson, 1970, 1971; Zuckerman, 1983, 1988; Zuckerman et al., 1964) and has been shown to play a major role in stimulus selection.

In developing an optimal level of arousal theory of the sensation-seeking motive, Zuckerman incorporated Berlyne's arousal potential qualities of stimulation and factors that reduce arousal potential, including repetition, constancy, and over-familiarity as ends of a sensation-seeking continuum.

According to this approach, individuals operate out of varying levels of physiological arousal, and therefore have differing needs for sensation. Those with lower arousal levels are referred to as high sensation seekers (HSS). It is thought that, in their attempts to elevate their physiological state, HSS almost continually need and seek out stimuli that are highly arousing. Conversely, low sensation seekers (LSS) operate out of a more comfortable level of arousal and tend to avoid stimuli that have the potential of pushing them beyond their existing physiological state. Thus, in general, the stimulus-hungry HSS prefers the excitement offered by novel, complex, and ambiguous stimuli, and the arousal-satiated LSS prefers things that he or she perceives as more familiar or less threatening.

Subsequent factor-analytic studies revealed four sensation-seeking factors and scales were constructed to measure them (Zuckerman, Eysenck, & Eysenck, 1978). As described by Zuckerman (1978, 1988) four dimensions of sensation seeking have been consistently observed:

1. Thrill and Adventure Seeking (TAS): A desire to seek sensation through physically risky activities which provide unusual situations and novel experiences (e.g., parachuting and scuba diving).

2. Experience Seeking (ES): A desire to seek sensation through a

nonconforming lifestyle, travel, music, art, drugs, and unconventional friends.

3. Disinhibition (DIS): A desire to seek sensation through social stimulation, parties, social drinking, and variety of sex partners.

4. Boredom Susceptibility (BS): An aversion to boredom produced by unchanging conditions or persons and a great restlessness when things are the same for any period of time.

Describing differences between high and low sensation seekers, Zuckerman (1988) observed that:

> The high sensation seeker is receptive to novel stimuli; the low tends to reject them, preferring the more familiar and less complex. The high sensation seeker's optimal level of stimulation may depend on the levels set by the characteristic level of arousal produced by novel stimuli. Anything producing lower arousal levels may be considered "boring." . . . Apart from the voluntary avoidance of high intensities of stimulation, the low sensation seeker may have a type of nervous system that reflects such stimulation or inhibits cortical reactivity to high intensity stimuli. (pp. 181–182)

There also is mounting evidence that Zuckerman's (1978) sensation-seeking scale taps fundamental biologically based dimensions of human behavior. This includes studies linking sensation seeking with monoanine oxidase (MAO), an enzyme that regulates the levels of monoamine neutrotransmitters in brain neurons (e.g., Murphy et al., 1977) and among males with levels of testosterone and estrogens (Fulker, Eysenck, & Zuckerman, 1980).

Our most recent study also found indirect evidence of this connection. Because of the strong relationship to hormonal changes, particularly to changes in testosterone levels, we should have expected levels of sensation seeking to increase with the onset of puberty, then to level out in the upper teens. Also, given that one of the principal changes involves testosterone, we should have observed somewhat higher scores among males. Tables 8.2 and 8.3 offer support for these expectations.

Activation Theory of Information Exposure

On the basis of the optimal level of arousal assumptions just described, an activation theory of information exposure was developed (Donohew et al., 1980) and tested in a number of studies (Donohew, 1981; Donohew & Coyle, 1988).

The theory assumes that part of the motivation for exposure to a

TABLE 8.2
SS Medians Among Junior High School
Students by Gender and Grade Level

Grade Level	All		Males		Females	
	N	SS Med.	N	SS Med.	N	SS Med.
7	403	17.7	199	18.3	204	17.0
8	395	20.5	193	21.7	202	18.4
9	426	21.3	211	22.9	215	20.3
All	1,224	19.8	603	20.9	621	18.4

TABLE 8.3
SS Medians Among Senior High School
Students by Gender and Grade Level

Grade Level	All		Males		Females	
	N	SS Med.	N	SS Med.	N	SS Med.
10	372	20	157	21	215	18
11	324	20	137	20	187	19
12	209	20	78	22	131	19
All	905	20	372	21	533	19

message involves need for stimulation rather than cognitive need for information alone (Donohew, Finn, & Christ, 1988; Finn, 1985a, 1985b). It holds that consistency seeking and variety seeking are two ends of a single continuum and offers propositions about information exposure based on activation needs.

Donohew and associates proposed (Fig. 8.1) that individuals enter information-exposure situations with the expectation of achieving or maintaining an optimal state of activation. It should be noted, however, that the monitoring of this "expectation" may be carried out at a low level of awareness. If the level of activation significantly falls below or exceeds the optimal level, individuals will tend to turn away from the information and seek more or less exciting stimuli, as appropriate to their needs. If the activation level reaches or remains within some range perceived to be acceptable, individuals will continue to expose themselves to the information.

The activation model adds individual differences and an arousal-needs interpretation to the once widely accepted selective exposure hypothesis growing out of consistency theories (Christ, 1985; Fazio & Cooper, 1983; Maddi, 1968). Under that hypothesis (Festinger, 1964)

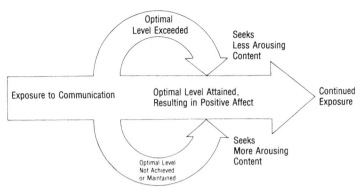

FIG. 8.1. An activation model of information exposure (reprinted from Donohue, Finn, & Christ, 1988).

individuals tend to seek information in an unbiased way when in a state of conflict, such as over a decision about to be made between alternatives of approximately equal attractiveness to them, or when in a state of postdecisional regret, when doubts arise about the wisdom of the option chosen. They avoid information when it conflicts with chosen alternatives about which they feel more certainty because such information causes the loss of equilibrium. Under the optimal level of arousal assumptions of the activation model, if this level of arousal exceeds the needs of the individual, he or she tends to turn away.

One shortcoming of this theory, however, is that it is difficult to specify just what is high arousal because there does not yet exist a parsimonious procedure for establishing individual arousal baselines. It is assumed that for high sensation-seeking individuals the most probable state at any given point in time is *stimulus hunger* and for low sensation seekers it is *stimulus satiation*. Thus, individuals with a high need for activation would most of the time be in an *arousal-seeking* mode and those with lower needs would be in an *arousal-avoidance* mode.

As noted elsewhere (Donohew, Finn, & Christ, 1988), the optimal level of arousal theory does not imply that individuals will read, watch, or listen to only those items which maintain arousal levels within desired boundaries:

> Although arousal needs do appear to guide them in their selections, they may choose to override these affective tugs for any of a number of reasons, such as desire to learn more about a topic of importance to them in which they perceive themselves to be deficient. (p. 195)

Recent research (Donohew, Helm, Cook, & Shatzer, 1987), suggests that *salience* of the message topic plays a key role in the type of processing to be conducted. Messages perceived to have high salience for subjects are likely to activate controlled processes, whereas under conditions of low salience (Donohew, 1982; Donohew et al., 1980), individuals are more likely to operate with low self-awareness or be guided by automatic processes. In either of the latter, arousal responses would be likely to play a greater role.

The most recent research was intended to test extensions of the theory in a drug-abuse prevention setting involving American teenagers ranging in age from 12 to 18 and to evaluate it as a model for use in public health campaigns. The study investigated not only the interaction of the arousal potential of two different message styles—narrative and expository—with individual arousal needs, but also the relationship between the content of the message and the degree to which individual receivers were personally involved with that content and their responses to it. Prior attitudes toward drug use also were measured.

In this study, we expected two of the groups to be guided by arousal needs and to respond more or less automatically: (a) individuals with high arousal needs who were already involved in drug use might turn away from the messages because they found that the messages describing the consequences of drug use were too discrepant with their attitudes and generated too much arousal; (b) individuals with low arousal needs who were not using drugs might find the material irrelevant and generate too little arousal to hold their attention.

The other two groups, individuals with high arousal needs not using drugs and those with low arousal needs who were using drugs were expected to be in a state of indecision about their behaviors and to respond according to cognitive needs (i.e., to prefer continued exposure to the messages).

The findings were consistent with these expectations. The study found significant interactions among the effects of activation needs (sensation seeking), involvement (marijuana use), and message style (narrative and expository) on preferences for continued exposure to messages about the effects of drug use. Style preferences varied by medium, print and television (see Fig. 8.2 and 8.3).

As predicted, subjects showing the greatest preferences for continued exposure to the message were those for whom it was perhaps most relevant to their behavior: subjects with low needs for activation (low sensation seekers) who were using marijuana and those with high needs who were not. The attitude measure verified that these two groups also were the most divided in their attitudes toward their behaviors, with 32.4% of low needs users and 21% of high needs nonusers holding attitudes counter to their behaviors.

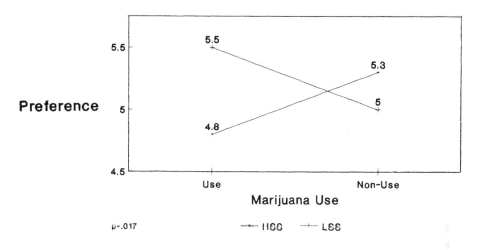

FIG. 8.2. Interaction of use and sensation seeking on preference.

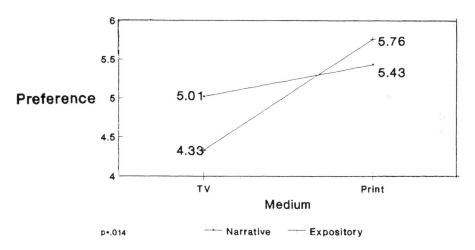

FIG. 8.3. Interaction of message style and medium on preference.

Also as predicted, nonusers with low arousal needs, those for whom
the message was least relevant, and users with high arousal needs,
those for whom the message was most discrepant, as the attitude measure was to verify, indicated the lowest preferences for continued exposure to the messages. These two groups were nearly unanimous in their
attitudes toward marijuana use. Over 96% of the low needs nonusers
were against it and, not far behind, 84% of the high needs users were
favorable to its use.

We also found support for predictions about arousal responses, comprehension, and other factors. In other words, we found that responses to the messages were not based on cognition alone, but on an interaction of biological (individual needs for arousal) and cognitive–behavioral factors, which we might assume defined salience for the individuals.

We decided to more formally incorporate the salience factor into our theory and test its effectiveness in a regression-based path analysis model (Joreskog & Sorbom, 1982). The model involves four variables: arousal and relevance as independent measures, and evaluation of the message and preferences to continue exposure as dependent measures.

The resulting model, found to significantly differ from a null model, indicates that the salience (cognitive) and arousal (affective) dimensions are unrelated and that their effects on the dependent measures are direct (see Fig. 8.4). Except as indicated, all relationships shown in the figure are statistically significant.

Arousal has a stronger relationship to both the dependent measures than does salience, continuing to support the arousal orientation of the existing theory but also adding support for inclusion of relevance as a separate dimension.

Other Research

Other researchers have supported an arousal needs approach to stimulus selection and information processing in various mass communication contexts (e.g., Bryant & Zillmann, 1984; Christ, 1985; Christ & Medoff, 1984; Fletcher, 1985). In addition, the activation model appears to have biological support, based on the findings that individuals are driven by the pleasure centers of the limbic system to continually search for stimulation (Martindale, 1981; Young, 1978). Thus, this approach to investigating selective responses to environmental stimuli can be assumed to be both theoretically and biologically grounded. As such, it has important implications for designers of communication messages in general and health communication messages in particular.

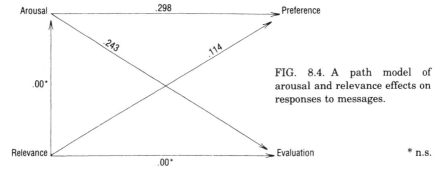

FIG. 8.4. A path model of arousal and relevance effects on responses to messages.

In light of this approach and the history of failed mass media campaigns seeking to change health behaviors on the basis of messages alone, our recommended approach to public health campaigns must necessarily be more complex.

We recommend a two-step process involving specially designed and targeted messages intended to motivate persons to call a hotline, then specially designed programs for subjects who call. Our approach to drug-abuse prevention campaigns has been to research and design separate messages to appeal to targeted subjects—in our instance high and low sensation seekers—and to offer separate appeals to each group. In the instance of the low sensation seekers, this has been an appeal to call a hotline to receive peer resistance skills training. For the high sensation seekers, it has been to call a hotline to learn about alternative activities providing sought-after stimulation in pro-social ways, as indicated by earlier research (Barnes & Olsen, 1977; Segal, Huba, & Singer, 1980; Zuckerman, 1983).

In this chapter, we have traced the connections previously described and have described evolution of a different kind of cybernetic system, one that is driven not only by cognitive responses to its environment, but also by physiological responses based in large part on whether the stimuli are novel or are ones to which the organism quickly habituates. In part, this arousal is generated by stimuli of direct concern to the individual, such as implications of information for his or her personal health.

REFERENCES

Bargh, J. A. (1984). Automatic and conscious processing of social information. In R. S. Wyer & T. K. Srull (Eds.), *Handbook of social cognition* (Vol. 3, pp. 1–44). Hillsdale, NJ: Lawrence Erlbaum Associates.

Bargh, J. A. (1988). Automatic information processing: Implications for communication and affect. In L. Donohew, H. Sypher, & T. Higgins, (Eds.), *Communication, social cognition and affect* (pp. 9–32). Hillsdale, NJ: Lawrence Erlbaum Associates.

Barnes, G. P., & Olsen, J. N. (1977). Usage patterns of non drug alternatives in adolescence. *Journal of Drug Education, 7,* 59–368.

Bates, M. E., Labouvier, E. W., & White, H. R. (n.d.). *The effect of sensation seeking needs on alcohol and marijuana use in adolescence.* Unpublished manuscript, Rutgers University, Center of Alcohol Studies, New Brunswick, NJ.

Berelson, B., Lazarsfeld, P., & McPhee, W. (1954). *Voting: A study of opinion formation in a presidential campaign.* Chicago: University of Chicago Press.

Berlyne, D. (1971). *Aesthetics and psychophysiology.* New York: Appleton-Century-Crofts.

Bryant, J., & Zillmann, D. (1984). Using television to alleviate boredom and stress:

Selective exposure as a function of induced excitational states. *Journal of Broadcasting, 28,* 1–20.

Cacioppo, J., & Petty, R. (1983). Foundations of social psychophysiology. In J. Cacioppo & R. Petty (Eds.), *Social psychophysiology: A sourcebook* (pp. 3–36). New York: Guilford.

Cacioppo, J., Petty, R., & Tassinary, L. (1988). Communication, social, cognition and affect: A psychophysiological approach. In L. Donohew, H. Sypher, & T. Higgins (Eds.), *Communication, social cognition and affect* (pp. 219–245). Hillsdale, NJ: Lawrence Erlbaum Associates.

Caplaces, R., & Starr, J. (1973). The negative message of anti-drug spots: Does it get across? *Public telecommunications review, 1,* 64–66.

Christ, W. (1985). The construct of arousal in communication research. *Human Communication Research, 11,* 575–592.

Christ, W., & Biggers, T. (1984). An exploratory investigation into the relationship between television program preference and emotion-eliciting qualities—a new theoretical perspective. *Western Journal of Speech Communication, 48*(3), 293–307.

Christ, W., & Medoff, N. J. (1984). Affective state and the selective exposure to and use of television. *Journal of Broadcasting, 28,* 51–63.

Delaney, R. W. (1978). *Comparison impact of two approaches to primary alcoholism prevention in Florida—1978.* Sarasota, FL: Department of Health and Rehabilitation Services, Alcohol Abuse Prevention Project.

Donohew, L. (1981). Arousal and affective responses to writing styles. *Journal of Applied Communication Research, 9,* 109–119.

Donohew, L. (1982). Newswriting styles: What arouses the reader? *Newspaper Research Journal, 3,* 3–6.

Donohew, L. (1988). *Effects of drug abuse message styles.* Final report on a study conducted under Grant No. DA03462 from the National Institute on Drug Abuse.

Donohew, L., & Coyle, K. (1988). *Getting past an ancient dragon: Reaching mass media audiences with information about public issues.* Paper presented at the 16th Conference and General Assembly, International Association for Mass Communication Research, Barcelona, Spain.

Donohew, L., Finn, S., & Christ, W. (1988). "The nature of news" revisited: The roles of affect, schemas, and cognition. In L. Donohew, H. Sypher, & T. Higgins (Eds.), *Communication, social cognition, and affect* (pp. 195–218). Hillsdale, NJ: Lawrence Erlbaum Associates.

Donohew, L., Helm, D. M., Cook, P. L., & Schatzer, M. J. (1987). *Sensation seeking, marijuana use, and responses to prevention messages: Implications for public health campaigns.* Paper presented at the meeting of the International Communication Association, Montreal.

Donohew, L., Palmgreen, P., & Duncan, J. (1980). An activation model of information exposure. *Communication Monographs, 47,* 295–303.

Donohew, L., Sypher, H., & Cook, P. (1988). Communication and affect: Themes and issues. *American Behavioral Scientist, 31*(3), 287–295.

Donohew, L., Sypher, H., & Higgins, T. (Eds.). (1988). *Communication, social cognition, and affect.* Hillsdale, NJ: Lawrence Erlbaum Associates.

Fazio, R., & Cooper, J. (1983). Arousal in the dissonance process. In J. Cacioppo & R. Petty (Eds.), *Social psychophysiology: A sourcebook* (pp. 122–152). New York: Guilford.

Festinger, L. (1964). *Conflict, decision, and dissonance.* Stanford, CA: Stanford University Press.

Finn, S. (1985a). Unpredictability as a correlate of reader enjoyment of news articles. *Journalism Quarterly, 62,* 334–339, 345.

Finn, S. (1985b). Information-theoretic measures of reader enjoyment. *Written Communication, 2,* 358–376.

Flay, B. (1986, May). *Mass media and smoking cessation.* Paper presented at a meeting of the International Communication Association convention, Chicago, IL.

Flay, B., DiTecco, D., & Schlegel, R. (1980). Mass media in health promotion: An analysis using an extended information-processing model. *Health Education Quarterly, 7,* 127–147.

Flay, B., & Sobel, J. L. (1983). The role of mass media in preventing adolescent substance abuse. In T. J. Glynn, C. G. Leukefeld, & J. P. Lundford (Eds.) *Preventing adolescent drug abuse: Intervention strategies.* NIDA Research Monograph Series (47).

Fletcher, J. (1985). Physiological responses to the media. In J. R. Dominick & J. Fletcher (Eds.), *Broadcasting research methods* (pp. 89–104). Boston: Allyn & Bacon.

Franklin, J., Donohew, L., Dhoundiyal, V., & Cook, P. (1988). Attention and our ancient past: the scaly thumb of the reptile. *American Behavioral Scientist, 31*(3), 312–326.

Fulker, D. W., Eysenck, S., & Zuckerman, M. (1980). A genetic and environmental analysis of sensation seeking. *Journal of Research in Personality, 14,* 261–281.

Hebb, D. C. (1955). Drives and the CNS (conceptual nervous system). *Psychological Review, 62,* 253–254.

Janis, I., & Feshbach, S. (1953). Effects of fear-arousing communications. *Journal of Abnormal and Social Psychology, 48,* 78–92.

Joreskog, K. G., & Sorbom, D. (1982). Recent developments in structural equation modeling. *Journal of Marketing Research, 9,* 404–416.

Klapper, J. (1960). *The effects of mass communication.* New York: The Free Press.

Langer, E. (1980). Rethinking the role of thought in social interaction. In H. Harvey, W. Ickes, & R. Kidd (Eds.), *New directions in attribution research* (Vol. 2, pp. 35–58). Hillsdale, NJ: Lawrence Erlbaum Associates.

Lazarsfeld, P., Berelson, B., & Gaudet, H. (1948). *The people's choice.* New York: Columbia University Press.

Lazarus, R. S. (1982). Thoughts on the relations between emotion and cognition. *American Psychologist, 37,* 1019–1024.

Luria, A. R. (1973). *The working brain.* New York: Basic Books.

Maddi, S. (1968). The pursuit of consistency and variety. In R. B. Abelson, E. Aronson, W. McGuire, T. Newcomb, M. Rosenberg, & P. Tannenbaum (Eds.), *Theories of cognitive consistency: A sourcebook* (pp. 267–274). Chicago, IL: Rand McNally.

Martindale, C. (1981). *Cognition and consciousness.* Homewood, IL: Dorsey.

Murphy, D. L., Belmaker, R. H., Buchsbaum, M. S., Martin, N. F., Ciaranello, R., & Wyatt, R. J. (1977). Biogenic amine related enzymes and personality variations in normals. *Psychological Medicine, 7,* 149–157.

Olds, M. E., & Fobes, J. L. (1981). The central basis of motivation: Intracranial self-stimulation studies. *Annual Review of Psychology, 32,* 523–574.

Pearson, P. (1970). Relationships between global and specified measures of novelty-seeking. *Journal of Consulting and Clinical Psychology, 37,* 23–30.

Pearson, P. (1971). Differential relationships of four forms of novelty experiencing. *Journal of Consulting and Clinical Psychology, 37,* 323–330.

Rappaport, M., Labow, P., & Williams, J. (1975). *The public evaluates the NIAAA public education campaign: A study for the U.S. department of health, education, and welfare, public health service, alcohol, drug abuse, and mental health administration* (2 vols.). Princeton, NJ: Opinion Research Corp.

Roloff, M. (1980). Self-awareness and the persuasion process: Do we really know what we are doing? In M. Roloff & G. Miller (Eds.), *Persuasion: New directions in theory and research* (pp. 29–66). Beverly Hills, CA: Sage.

Schank, R., & Abelson, R. (1977). *Scripts, plans, goals, and understanding: An inquiry into human knowledge structures.* Hillsdale, NJ: Lawrence Erlbaum Associates.

Schwarz, R. M., Burkhart, B. R., & Green, B. (1978). Turning on or turning off: Sensation seeking or tension reduction as motivational determinants of alcohol use. *Journal of Consulting and Clinical Psychology, 46,* 1144–1145.

Segal, B., Huba, G. J., & Singer, J. L. (1980). *Drugs, daydreaming and personality: A study of college youth.* Hillsdale, NJ: Lawrence Erlbaum Associates.

Segal, B., & Singer, J. L. (1976). Daydreaming, drug and alcohol use in college students: A factor analytic study. *Addictive Behaviors, 1,* 227–235.

Shiffrin, R., & Schneider, W. (1977). Controlled and automatic information processing, II: Perceptual learning, automatic attending, and a general theory. *Psychological Review, 84,* 127–190.

Wundt, W. (1874). *Grundzuge der physiologischen Psychologie* [Principles of physiological psychology]. Leipzig: Englemann.

Yerkes, R. M., & Dodson, J. D. (1908). The relation of strength of stimulus to rapidity of habit formation. *Journal of Comparative and Neurological Psychology, 18,* 459–482.

Young, J. Z. (1978). *Programs of the brain.* London: Oxford University Press.

Zajonc, R. B. (1968). Cognitive theories in social psychology. In G. Lindsey & E. Aronson (Eds.), *The handbook of social psychology* (2nd ed., pp. 320–411). Reading, MA: Addison-Wesley.

Zajonc, R. B. (1980). Feeling and thinking: Preferences need no inferences. *American Psychologist, 39,* 117–123.

Zajonc, R. B. (1984). On the primacy of affect. *American Psychologist, 39,* 117–123.

Zillmann, D. (1988a). Mood management: Using entertainment to full advantage. In L. Donohew, H. Sypher, & T. Higgins (Eds.), *Communication, social cognition and affect* (pp. 147–171). Hillsdale, NJ: Lawrence Erlbaum Associates.

Zillmann, D. (1988b). Mood management through communication choices. *American Behavioral Scientist, 31*(3), 327–340.

Zillmann, D., & Bryant, J. (1985). Affect, mood and emotion as determinants of selective exposure. In D. Zillmann & J. Bryant (Eds.), *Selective exposure to communication* (pp. 157–180). Hillsdale, NJ: Lawrence Erlbaum Associates.

Zuckerman, M. (1978). *Sensation seeking: Beyond the optimal level of arousal.* Hillsdale, NJ: Lawrence Erlbaum Associates.

Zuckerman, M. (1983). *Biological bases of sensation seeking, impulsivity and anxiety.* Hillsdale, NJ: Lawrence Erlbaum Associates.

Zuckerman, M. (1988). Behavior and biology: Research on sensation seeking and reactions to the media. In L. Donohew, H. Sypher, & E. T. Higgins (Eds.), *Communication, social cognition, and affect* (pp. 173–194). Hillsdale, NJ: Lawrence Erlbaum Associates.

Zuckerman, M., Eysenck, S., & Eysenck, H. J. (1978). Sensation seeking in England and America: Cross-cultural, age and sex comparisons. *Journal of Consulting and Clinical Psychology, 46,* 139–149.

Zuckerman, M., Kolin, E. A., Price, L., & Zoob, I. (1964). Development of a sensation-seeking scale. *Journal of Consulting Psychology, 28,* 477–482.

9

Public Health Campaigns:
Mass Media Strategies

Jane D. Brown
University of North Carolina

Edna F. Einsiedel
University of Calgary

The mass media have been used in health promotion efforts for many years. Television, radio, newspapers, magazines, billboards, posters, and pamphlets have been used to encourage people to fasten seatbelts (Robertson et al., 1974), to quit smoking (Flay, 1987a), to use contraceptives (Udry, 1974), and most recently, to "just say no" to drugs and to use condoms to protect against the spread of the AIDS virus (Backer, 1988). Although many public health educators (and mass communication researchers) remain somewhat pessimistic about the potential of the mass media to effect long-term changes in behavior, most would now agree that the mass media can be effective in increasing awareness of health issues. The mass media also can be effective in stimulating attitude and behavior change, especially if media messages are supplemented with interpersonal and community structures that support such changes. (For reviews of mass media health campaigns, see Atkin, 1979; Flay, 1987a; Lau, Kane, Berry, Ware, & Roy, 1980; Solomon, 1982.)

Today, a number of organizations and institutions are using the mass media as part of their health education efforts, especially when potential audiences are large and widely dispersed. Although comprehensive evaluations of these efforts are scarce, those that have been conducted show that the most effective media campaigns are based on a thorough understanding of the health issue and the audience or audiences to be reached. Effective campaigns have reached specific audiences with appropriate media and consistent messages based on extensive pretesting and often the mass media messages have been supplemented with some form of face-to-face or interpersonal communication (Rogers & Storey, 1987). Health educators have begun to learn that effective use of the mass media requires planning, research, and consideration of the environment in which the media are used.

This chapter discusses some general guidelines that should be considered as public health strategies that include the mass media are developed. We discuss these guidelines within a series of five steps that usually are taken as a media campaign is designed and implemented. A number of these guidelines are drawn from experience in what is now called "social marketing." This approach, originally articulated in the early 1970s (Kotler & Zaltman, 1971), borrows lessons learned by commercial product advertisers and applies them to social issues. It now has been applied extensively to a variety of health issues (Manoff, 1985).

The social marketing approach focuses attention on the audience and its social, political, and economic environment. From this perspective, campaign planners are compelled to consider not only what it is they are really trying to get people to do, but also why the audience might be motivated to comply with or might resist engaging in the desired behavior. At each step in the campaign process, from defining the problem and establishing realistic objectives, to message design and media planning and implementation, the needs, motivations, and resources of the audience are considered. Existing data, interviews with small groups and surveys of samples of the potential audience are used to learn more about the audience and its environment. Whenever possible, existing structures such as smoking cessation clinics and support groups or rules and regulations that can supplement the media campaign are utilized. Although marketers rarely discuss the theoretical rationale of these principles of marketing, social scientific theories of learning undergird most of them (Einsiedel & Cochrane, 1988).

STEPS IN CONDUCTING A MASS MEDIA
PUBLIC HEALTH CAMPAIGN

Define Problem and Set Objectives

The first step in any health campaign should be to develop a clear definition of the problem to be discussed and to set realistic objectives based on this problem definition. This is not always as easy as it sounds. Often the difficulty lies in knowing where in the persuasion process the campaign should be aimed. Typically, it has been assumed that in order to persuade people to do something, we first must make them aware of the issue and then give them facts about the side of the issue we are promoting (and perhaps counter-arguments about other sides of the issue). Presumably, the individual then will change his or her attitudes about the issue and subsequently, will adopt the desired behavior (Bettinghaus, 1986).

Two factors complicate this scenario. First, results from previous mass media campaigns show that the mass media are most effective at the early stages in this process—they are best at increasing public awareness of health issues and they can provide facts that lead to increased knowledge about the issue. The media also may be able to stimulate interpersonal communication and some immediate action such as calling a hotline for more information, but in general, the media, especially in isolation from other kinds of reinforcement, will not be very effective in generating long-term changes in deep-seated attitudes and ingrained behaviors (Rogers & Storey, 1987).

Second, the knowledge–attitude–behavior continuum does not always work in this order (Bettinghaus, 1986). People do sometimes change behavior without previous change in attitudes, especially when adoption of the new behavior is inexpensive or convenient or when they have little alternative. For example, people are more likely to fasten their seat belts or refrain from cigarette smoking when compelled to by law (Milio, 1986).

Obviously, then, the campaign planner must be thoroughly aware of the nature of the health issue with which he or she is dealing, must know where the majority of the potential audience is in the persuasion process, and to what extent existing regulations and structures augment desired outcomes. This understanding will directly influence how the problem is defined and how the media are used.

Health officials in New York City working to stem the spread of the AIDS virus among intravenous drug users, for example, initially believed that their education campaigns should focus on increasing awareness of the dangers of the virus and knowledge of how it was spread. A mass media campaign was developed to run on radio stations with greatest reach in areas of the city with the highest rates of drug users. Outreach workers soon realized, however, that most needle users already were aware of the dangers of the virus and knew they should not be sharing dirty needles. The problem had very quickly become one of motivating a very hard-to-reach population to change a deeply ingrained ritual of needle sharing. Health officials, realizing that the mass media probably were going to be much less effective in helping to solve the problem of dirty needles, renewed efforts to expand outreach programs that included interpersonal support for the use of clean needles, or preferably, kicking the drug habit altogether. This new definition of the problem also pointed to the need to change existing laws so that clean needles could be distributed without prescriptions and focused attention on the need for increased access to drug rehabilitation programs (Perry, 1988).

Setting Campaign Objectives. Once the problem has been defined adequately, realistic campaign objectives should be established. These objectives should be specific, achievable and measurable (Maccoby & Solomon, 1981). Setting objectives allows planners to develop an overall campaign strategy and a budget. Objectives also establish the standard by which the success of the campaign can be measured (Kotler, 1982). Campaign planners should not be afraid to set objectives that may at first seem trivial. Although some critics have argued that previous media campaigns were failures because they accounted for less than 10 percent of the variance in a health behavior, others have pointed out that even such an apparently small change can be quite dramatic across the large audiences often reached by the mass media (Warner, 1987).

Identify Target Audiences

A key element in social marketing is "market segmentation." Segmentation of the potential audience for the media campaign allows planners to focus on the most appropriate segments of the audience and to study the behavior of each segment in order to identify the most cost-effective marketing strategies (Kotler, 1982). Audience segmentation often involves the use of existing research in an effort to learn as much as possible about potential audiences and the individual or structural factors that influence each audience segment's current health behaviors. When little is known about the audience segment, new studies should be conducted. Such research usually is called *formative research* because it is used to formulate the rest of the campaign (Flay, 1987b).

In the early 1980s, for example, the U.S. National Cancer Institute, given the goal of halving the number of cancer deaths in the country by the year 2000, funded intervention projects designed to reach various audience segments including health practitioners (physicians and dentists), minority groups, women, and adolescents. These groups were targeted because previous research had shown that health practitioners might be effective in getting their patients to quit smoking, and because minority group members, women, and adolescents were still at high risk of becoming cigarette smokers (National Institutes of Health, 1983).

As part of this effort, a team of public health and communication specialists at the University of North Carolina developed a set of mass media campaigns aimed at young adolescents who had not yet begun to smoke cigarettes (Bauman et al., 1988). The adolescent audience was segmented into two groups: those who had begun to smoke and those who had not. Previous research showed that most smokers began smoking between the ages of 15 and 19. Thus, a set of messages were developed aimed at the segment that had not yet begun to smoke (12- to 15-year-olds) with the long-term goal of keeping a small portion of this market segment from becoming cigarette smokers. Given the findings of other communication campaigns, the planners reasoned that the mass media probably would be more effective in reinforcing the existing behavior of not smoking than they would be in convincing people to give up the habit once they had started.

In Alberta, Canada, a four-community cancer prevention program has focused on five cancer types: lung, colon, cervix, breast and skin. Previous research was used to identify certain groups at risk for each cancer type. Two segments of women were identified as appropriate target audiences for messages about prevention and early detection of breast cancer. Messages encouraging regular mammograms were designed for women over 50 at higher than average risk. Early detection was promoted among younger females by encouraging regular breast self-examinations and physical examinations by a health professional.

These examples illustrate some of the basic principles of market segmentation. Campaign planners should first decide which audiences are most appropriately addressed by the campaign, given the established problem and objectives. Often public health officials will want to choose audience segments that are at greatest risk of either adopting the unhealthy behavior or suffering from it. Planners then need to know why the segment (or segments) adopts the behavior or persists in it. At this point, campaign planners may use a number of theories of human behavior to guide them in developing successful persuasion strategies. The Stanford health interventions, for example, are based to a large extent on Bandura's (1977) social learning theory; the North Carolina team's campaigns were based on conceptualizations of human behavior that propose that people behave to maximize positive consequences and to minimize the negative consequences of their behavior (Fishbein & Ajzen, 1975).

The planner also must consider the extent to which the targeted audience segment (or segments) is confronted with competing messages. Health campaigns often are launched in hostile media environments (Wallack, 1981). In the United States, tobacco and alcohol companies spend millions of dollars promoting cigarette smoking and alcohol consumption. Advertisements for fast foods high in fat and sugar permeate all forms of the mass media. Unhealthy behavior often is portrayed as convenient, fun, youthful and/or glamorous in these advertisements as well as in entertainment programming (Gerbner, Morgan, & Signorielli, 1982).

Some campaigns have been designed expressly to counter some of the implicit and explicit claims in such media content. Warner (1977, 1981) has shown, for example, that the counter-advertising aired in the days before the ban on cigarette advertising on television and radio, was effective in reducing cigarette consumption and, at the least, was instrumental in convincing the tobacco companies that they should suffer the ban rather than be subjected to counter-argument in the same medium (Warner, 1979). But public health institutions rarely have the resources to mount campaigns as far-reaching as those of major product advertisers.

Wallack (1981, 1984) and others (Milio, 1986) argue that mass media campaigns aimed only at affecting individual health habits may be misdirected and certainly will not have long-term effects unless they are conducted in environments that encourage and support healthy behavior. What good does it do, for example, to tell people they should eat less fatty food when that is all they can get at the grocery store or at their local restaurant? What good does it do to ask people to not drive a car after drinking alcohol when alcohol is as easy to get at the gas station as gasoline?

A few health campaigns have taken such questions seriously. As part of the Minnesota Heart Health Program's (MHHP) community intervention (Blackburn et al., 1983) to reduce cardiovascular risk factors, for example, restaurants were encouraged to provide low-fat entrees that then were designated by red hearts on their menus and promoted in media advertisements. In North Karelia, Finland, the media health campaign promoting the reduction of cardiovascular risk factors was augmented by government subsidies for low-fat milk products (Puska et al., 1979).

Other kinds of actions aimed at changing the "opportunity structure" for healthy behaviors have included what are sometimes called *engineering* and *enforcement solutions* (Paisley, 1981). The installation of airbags in new cars is one example of an engineering solution to the problem of drivers being unwilling to buckle their seatbelts. A law that levies a fine for not buckling seatbelts is an enforcement solution. Campaign planners should consider how their education strategies might be supplemented or enhanced by concomitant changes in technology and rules and regulations. These, of course, often will be difficult alternatives, especially if they threaten existing economic or power structures or raise questions of individual choice (Wallack, 1984). We need only consider, for example, how long it has taken to regulate cigarette smoking in public places. Nevertheless, campaign planners should consider whether resources can be directed at changing the unhealthy system as well as at unhealthy individuals in the system. At the very least, planners should work on providing increased opportunities for individuals to engage in the desired healthy behaviors at low psychological and financial cost.

Choose Appropriate Influence Channels

Once target audience segments have been identified, appropriate "influence channels" (Kotler, 1982) can be chosen. Influence channels are the means by which "materials" (Manoff, 1985) are transmitted to individuals in the targeted audience. As can be seen in Table 9.1, a variety of media influence channels are available for transmitting a variety of materials. Each kind of channel has advantages and disadvantages in terms of cost and ability to segment the audience. Materials differ in terms of the extent to which the source has control over message content and what Manoff (1985) called "media values"— communication attributes such as color, sight, and sound. In general, campaign planners try to use multiple channels and multiple materials in the interest of reaching as much of the audience as frequently as possible.

TABLE 9.1
Media Influence Channels and Materials

Media Influence Channel	Materials
Television broadcast cable videocassettes	• Public service announcements (PSAs) • Paid advertisements • News stories, features on issue with health professionals • Themes in entertainment programming • Educational programs
Radio	• PSAs, paid advertisements • News and feature stories • Themes in songs
Magazines	• PSAs, paid advertisements • News and feature stories
Newspapers	• PSAs, paid advertisements • News and feature stories
Direct mail	• Brochures, pamphlets
Telephone	• Hotlines for counseling, referral

In the antismoking campaigns, for example, advertising time was bought on radio stations popular with young adolescents, on the music television (MTV) channel in local markets, and in afternoon and Saturday morning broadcast television programming (Bauman et al., 1988). Audience research showed that adolescents were infrequent readers of newspapers but were avid radio listeners. MTV was an especially attractive influence channel not only because it attracted a large portion of the adolescent audience, but also because it was much less expensive to purchase advertising time on cable than on broadcast television channels.

Paid advertising, although expensive, allows the campaign planner control over message content and timing. Broadcasters are notorious for running public service announcements (PSAs) at times when all but the most recalcitrant insomniacs are asleep. Media scholars have suggested that a number of campaigns have been ineffective because the audience simply did not see the messages (Flay, 1981; O'Keefe & Reid-Nash, 1986). PSAs can be effective, however, especially if they are of high quality and local organizations are used to encourage local radio and television stations and newspapers to use them (Maloney & Hersey, 1984). Recent experience with antismoking campaigns in Minnesota and Vermont also suggests that television stations may donate free time when some advertising time is bought (Minnesota Institute of Public Health, 1988; Worden et al., 1988).

If possible, media channels should be supplemented with interpersonal contact of some sort. In general, interpersonal or nonmediated channels are more effective in delivering complex, emotionally volatile, and persuasive messages and in inducing complex behavior change, provided that the source is perceived as credible. They also are effective when there is a small, selective audience and when control over the presentation of the material is required (Rogers, 1973a).

Media campaigns have been conducted in concert with public meetings, workshops, phone calls, staged events, and demonstrations. The North Carolina team's antismoking campaigns included a direct mail component that encouraged adolescents to sign up their friends to enter a nonsmoker sweepstakes (Bauman et al., 1988). The American AIDS education campaign included a booklet sent to every household that encouraged recipients to "read this brochure and talk about it with those you love" ("U.S. will mail AIDS advisory to all households," 1988). Telephone counseling has been an important part of the AIDS education efforts across the country because it allows for confidential discussion of sensitive topics that traditionally have been off limits for public (and media) discussion (Brown, Waszak, & Childers, in press).

Develop Materials and Messages

Whether an audience receives, listens to, understands, remembers, and responds to campaign materials largely depends on five aspects of the message presentation: content appeal, style, frequency, timing, and accessibility (Atkin, 1981; Bettinghaus, 1986; Rogers & Storey, 1987). Messages must be presented frequently and in the media the targeted audience is likely to attend to. The most effective content appeals are those that have been designed specifically to fit the audience, channel, source, topic, and intended effect, based on formative research. Appeals should be relevant to individuals in the target audience. Uses and gratifications research shows that it is difficult for receivers to justify the time and effort required to process a message unless the message somehow gratifies their need for knowledge or assists them in solving a problem that affects their lives (Atkin, 1981; Dervin, 1981). Research in cognitive psychology shows that the format of materials is important in leading to comprehension and recall of central message elements (Stewart, 1986).

The design and testing of materials and messages is a central part of formative research—campaign planners need to develop messages that attract the audience's attention, are understandable and will motivate the audience to respond in the desired manner. One of the most relevant strategies for message design has been developed by the U.S. National Institutes of Health (1982) and described in a publication called *Pretesting in Health Communications*. This plan for pretesting of messages includes assessing the readability of printed materials and conducting interviews with individuals and small groups to assess comprehension, recall, personal relevance, and controversial elements in proposed messages. Manoff (1985) developed a "resistance resolution model" of message design that points to the need for searching out "resistance points" to change. From this perspective, messages can be designed to address an individual's reasons for not wanting to comply with the behavior advocated in the message.

This approach was taken in developing the messages for the anti-smoking campaigns aimed at adolescent nonsmokers. Bauman (Bauman & Chenoweth, 1984; Bauman, Fisher, Bryan, & Chenoweth, 1984) had identified 52 positive and negative consequences that adolescents associated with cigarette smoking. Subsequent analyses showed that seven underlying themes (including such negative expected consequences as having bad breath, losing friends, and getting into trouble with adults, and such positive expected consequences as having fun and being relaxed) were significant predictors of adolescent smoking. These seven themes were then used as core concepts for message development. In 30-second radio and television spots young adolescents talked about how they had made decisions not to smoke because they had found that negative outcomes were more likely than positive ones.

One of the most extensively studied aspects of persuasion is source credibility. A number of studies generally support the intuitive notion that people are more likely to agree with a message and perhaps follow its requests if they find the source or spokesperson trustworthy, competent, and attractive (Atkin, 1979). Again, formative research can help planners determine which sources are perceived as credible by the targeted audience. In the antismoking campaigns, for example, a series of focus group interviews and interviews in schools showed that adolescents, contrary to expectations, found a slightly deviant look less credible than the look of an average, slightly older, self-confident adolescent. They, in effect, confirmed what Rogers (1973b) called "source homophily"—in general, people are more likely to be persuaded by people seen as similar to themselves.

Implement and Evaluate

As a consequence of political pressures, resource constraints, and the simple need to know whether program objectives are met, program evaluation has become an indispensable component of health education campaigns. It is an ongoing activity that provides continuous feedback about how the campaign is doing. We already have discussed how formative research is conducted in the early phases of the campaign planning process. What is usually described as "summative evaluation" is conducted once the media messages have been developed and the media plan implemented.

Why Have a Summative Evaluation?   An evaluation component is included in a communication campaign for very practical reasons. The first reason is accountability. Many government agencies and other donor organizations that fund health communication programs naturally are interested in answering the question: "Did it work?" Responses to this question also have important practical implications for program replication and generalizability. Campaign planners need to know if the program should be repeated or revised, and if it could be used in other situations. Finally, evaluation allows the organization that sponsors the media campaign to gauge its own efficiency and effectiveness, to monitor whether objectives are achieved and to establish new objectives.

What to Evaluate. Given these reasons for evaluation, two broad areas usually are considered in designing summative evaluations. Evaluations should include both an assessment of the campaign process and the effects or impact of the campaign. In community-based campaigns it also is important to assess the "social relevance" of the campaign. There are essentially three questions that need to be answered here: (a) What effects should be measured? (b) With which methods should they be measured? and (c) For what purpose? Obviously, the answers to all three questions are inextricably linked.

The first question is important for both heuristic and policy reasons. Because many campaigns have objectives of changing individual unhealthy behaviors to healthier ones (e.g., consumption of polyunsaturated fat and reduction of alcohol, cigarette smoking, drunk driving), most campaign planners, from a policy perspective, would like to be able to show that the campaign caused an increase in healthy behavior among the targeted audience. On the other hand, as we have discussed previously, given that the mass media probably are more effective in the earlier stages of the persuasion process (i.e., increasing awareness and knowledge), evaluators often have to be satisfied with assessing changes in awareness and knowledge rather than behavior.

The theoretical model guiding the campaign also will influence which effects are examined. Campaigns based on the health-belief model (Rosenstock, 1974), for example, assume a sequence of changes beginning with: (a) awareness of a problem and leading to (b) increased knowledge (including an understanding of susceptibility to a disease and the consequences of illness), (c) increased motivation as a result of an evaluation of the benefits of action and the risks of inaction that all finally lead to (d) the performance of the healthy behavior. Such a model obviously specifies the types of effects to be measured.

If campaign objectives have been specified appropriately, theoretical needs and policy imperatives should converge. In the case of educational campaigns about AIDS, for example, campaign objectives have included awareness and knowledge as well as behavioral change among the populations at high risk. These campaigns have been important in helping to change the public's knowledge and beliefs about such issues as the need for confidential testing, continued employment of people with the HIV virus, and allowing children with AIDS to stay in school.

The problem of appropriate evaluation methods has been treated in detail elsewhere (see, e.g., Flay, 1987b; Flay & Cook, 1981; Lau et al., 1980). We simply want to emphasize that the choice of measurement approaches is dependent on the relative importance of three factors: policy relevance, cost, and whether documentation of a causal sequence is required. Flay and Cook (1981) described three commonly used paradigms for measuring effects that vary on each of these three factors. This is summarized in Table 9.2.

The *advertising* approach involves the use of surveys of random samples of the target audience or specific subgroups of the target audience. Such a survey might include a range of questions from awareness and recall of specific messages to knowledge about campaign issues, attitudes, and self-reported behaviors, but the focus usually is on message recall and recognition. Advertisers often equate message recall with persuasion and hence often do not worry about measuring actual behavior. The advertising approach also does not include the use of control groups or surveys taken both before and after the campaign. It thus is not suited for establishing whether or not the campaign changed the audience in any way. The primary advantage of the approach is that one-shot surveys can be conducted relatively inexpensively.

The *monitoring* approach calls for tracking information requests or program enrollments that occur as a result of media presentations. Evaluations of this sort have included monitoring cigarette and alcohol sales, the incidence of accidents caused by drunk drivers, and the sale of fruits, vegetables, and lean meat. This approach, although inexpensive, neglects lower order effects such as awareness and knowledge gain, however, and it is difficult to say with certainty that changes in such behavioral indicators were caused by the media campaign and not by other trends in the environment. Ideally, these other trends should be assessed throughout the campaign process.

The *experimental* approach involves the comparison of groups exposed to the campaign (or various kinds of campaigns) with groups that have not been exposed (called *control groups*). The Stanford three-city study (Maccoby & Solomon, 1981), for example, evaluated the effects of a campaign that included messages presented only in the media with a campaign that used both media and interpersonal communication. Measures of healthy behaviors were taken both before and after the campaigns and in another city that had received neither health campaign.

TABLE 9.2
Relative Cost Benefits for Evaluation Approaches

	Evaluation Approaches		
	Advertising	*Monitoring*	*Experimental*
Causal inference	Low	Low	High
Policy relevance	Low	High	High
Cost	Low	Low	High

The experimental approach, although providing the most valid test of causality, is expensive because it requires that surveys be conducted both before and after the media campaign and/or that surveys be conducted in a comparable population that did not receive the campaign. From a policy perspective, it also may be unfeasible or even unethical to designate some segment of the population as a control group, especially when the campaign includes information that may save lives. It would have been very difficult for the American government, for example, to have decided that part of the country should not receive booklets on how to prevent the spread of the virus that causes AIDS just so they could test the effectiveness of the literature.

Process Evaluation. Another important question to answer is why the program worked or did not work. It is a rare campaign in which all program materials and strategies are successful in achieving their objectives. Process evaluation assists in identifying which elements of the campaign worked and provides documentation of temporal sequence and the mix of resources employed. Campaign managers should be able to answer the following kinds of questions:

- What materials were prepared? Did the materials reach their target audiences? Were they understood? Were they used as intended?
- Did channels selected present materials as planned? If PSAs were used, when and how often were they aired?
- Did the targeted audiences participate in prescribed activities? Did they engage in all of them and at the appropriate times?
- What organizational/community resources were expended, when, and for how long?

Providing documentation for these activities is both easy and difficult. The easy part is listing the activities, materials, resources, timelines, and so forth. The difficult part is verifying what actually occurred. With limited resources, the evaluator may have to limit documentation to priority activities.

Another aspect of process evaluation is what we call *environmental* documentation or establishing what else occurred in the audience's environment that might have affected its health behaviors during the campaign period. For some programs, especially those without randomly assigned control and treatment areas, this documentation is particularly important. The Steve Fonyo Cancer Prevention Program in Alberta, Canada (Birdsell, McGregor, & Leinweber, 1988), for instance, has tracked such things as the number of weight-loss and quit-smoking clinics and the frequency of stories about nutrition, health, cancer, and fitness in the newspapers in their study communities. This will help them sort out the effects of their campaign from the effects of efforts generated by other groups and media in the community. Table 9.3 shows examples of some of the kinds of documentation that can be used in internal and environmental process evaluations.

Evaluation of Social Relevance.   This is the area probably least often considered for evaluation. It is presented as an evaluation area because of increasing interest in the participative model of health education promotion and delivery. This model, which has been adopted by the World Health Organization (1983), encourages community involvement in the process of planning and implementation of health education programs. Both the Steve Fonyo Cancer Prevention Program and the Minnesota Heart Health Program have included their targeted communities in the development of their media-based campaigns.

The evaluation of social relevance requires the combination of effects and process evaluation with a focus on the assessment of impact at the community level. Such questions as the following would need to be answered: How much community participation was elicited and at what stages? What are citizens' perceptions of the value of the program to the community as a whole (in contrast to perceived effects on themselves as individuals)? Have community norms been changed as a result of the campaign? Were existing community organizations and structures used in various phases of the program?

According to organizers of the Minnesota program, the community task forces established to assist in strategic planning contributed to

TABLE 9.3
Documentation Used in Internal and Environmental
Process Evaluations

Internal/Program	*External/Environmental*
• Attendance/enrollment records	• Records of grocery store sales, restaurant menu choices
• Program call-ins	• Media coverage of related health issues
• Phone calls for info. and referral	• Social statistics about health status
• Direct-mail response information	• Community activities that might have impact on program objectives
• Program logs	
• Participation rates in program delivery (e.g., number of volunteers)	

"the energy and commitment necessary to implement heart health programs in the community, and the development of a social environment and community norms supportive of heart health" (Carlaw, Mittlemark, Bracht, & Luepker, 1984). Similarly, community involvement in the Alberta cancer risk reduction program has been positive (Birdsell, McGregor, & Leinweber, 1988).

CONCLUSION

The mass media might be seen most appropriately as another set of tools that can be used to promote desirable public policies and healthy individual behaviors. Although not a grand panacea for the problems of unhealthy lifestyles and the policies that support them, the mass media, if used appropriately, can play an important role in moving us closer to better health for all. Effective use of the mass media requires thoughtful planning and goal setting, a clear understanding of the health issue and the audience, and continuing assessment of what works and does not work.

ACKNOWLEDGMENT

The first author would like to thank the Gannett Center for Media Studies for providing generous space and time to work on this chapter.

REFERENCES

Atkin, C. K. (1979). Research evidence on mass mediated health communication campaigns: In D. Nimmo (Ed.), *Communication yearbook III* (pp. 655–668). New Brunswick, NJ: Transaction Books.

Atkin, C. K. (1981). Mass media information campaign effectiveness: In R. E. Rice & W. J. Paisley (Eds.), *Public communication campaigns* (pp. 265–279). Beverly Hills, CA: Sage.

Backer, T. E. (1988). Health professionals' and mass media's campaigns to prevent AIDS and drug abuse. *Counseling and Human Development, 20*(7), 2–10.

Bandura, A. (1977). *Social learning theory.* Englewood Cliffs, NJ: Prentice-Hall.

Bauman, K. E., Brown, J. D., Bryan, E. S., Fisher, L. A., Padgett, C. A., Sweeney, J. M. (1988). Three mass media campaigns to prevent adolescent cigarette smoking. *Preventive Medicine, 17,* 510–530.

Bauman, K. E., & Chenoweth, R. L. (1984). The relationship between the consequences adolescents expect from smoking and their behavior: A factor analysis with panel data. *Journal of applied social psychology, 14,* 28–41.

Bauman, K. E., Fisher, L. A., Bryan, E. S., & Chenoweth, R. L. (1984). Antecedents, subjective expected utility, and behavior: A panel study of adolescent cigarette smoking. *Addictive Behaviors, 9,* 121–136.

Bettinghaus, E. P. (1986). Health promotion and the knowledge-attitude-behavior continuum. *Preventive Medicine, 15*(5), 475–491.

Birdsell, J., McGregor, E., & Leinweber, C. (1988). *Steve Fonyo Cancer Prevention Program: Progress report.* Unpublished manuscript, Alberta Cancer Board, Calgary, Alberta.

Blackburn, H. W., Luepker, R. V., Kline, F. G., Bracht, N., Carlaw, R., Jacobs, D., Mittelmark, M., Stauffer, L., & Taylor, H. L. (1983). The Minnesota Heart Health Program: A research and demonstration project in cardiovascular disease prevention: In S. Weiss (Ed.), *Settings for health promotion in behavioral health: A handbook for health enhancement and disease prevention* (pp. 1171–1178). Silver Spring, MD: Wiley.

Brown, J. D., Waszak, C. S., & Childers, K. W. (in press). Sexuality and communication campaigns: In C. Salmon (Ed.), *Information campaigns: Managing the process of social change.* Beverly Hills, CA: Sage.

Carlaw, R. W., Mittlemark, M. B., Bracht, N., & R. Luepker (1984). Organization for a community cardiovascular health program: Experiences from the Minnesota Heart Health Program. *Health education quarterly, 11*(3), 243–252.

Dervin, B. (1981). Mass communicating: Changing conceptions of the audience: In R. E. Rice & W. J. Paisley (Eds.), *Public communication campaigns* (pp. 71–87). Beverly Hills, CA: Sage.

Einsiedel, E., & Cochrane, K. (1988). *Using social marketing and theoretical perspectives for health campaigns to adolescents.* Paper presented at annual conference of the International Communication Association, New Orleans, LA.

Fishbein, M., & Ajzen, I. (1975). *Belief, attitude, intention, and behavior: An introduction to theory and research.* Reading, MA: Addison-Wesley.

Flay, B. R. (1981). On improving the chances of mass media health promotion programs causing meaningful changes in behavior: In M. Meyer (Ed.), *Health education by television and radio: Contributions to an international conference with a selected bibliography* (pp. 56–89). Munchen: K. G. Saur.

Flay, B. R. (1987a). Mass media and smoking cessation: A critical review. *American Journal of Public Health, 77*(2), 153–160.

Flay, B. R. (1987b). Evaluation of the development, dissemination and effectiveness of mass media health programming. *Health education research, 2*(2), 123–129.

Flay, B. R., & Cook, R. D. (1981). Evaluation of mass media prevention campaigns: In R. E. Rice & W. J. Paisley (Eds.), *Public communication campaigns* (pp. 239–264). Beverly Hills, CA: Sage.

Gerbner, G., Morgan, M., & Signorielli, N. (1982). Programming health portrayals: What viewers see, say, and do: In D. Pearl, L. Bouthilet, & J. Lazar (Eds.), *Television and behavior: Ten years of scientific progress and implications for the Eighties* (pp. 291–307). Rockville, MD: National Institute of Mental Health.

Kotler, P. (1982). *Marketing for nonprofit organizations.* Englewood Cliffs, NJ: Prentice-Hall.

Kotler, P., & Zaltman, G. (1971). Social marketing: An approach to planned social change. *Journal of marketing, 35,* 3–12.

Lau, R., Kane, R., Berry, S., Ware, J., & Roy, D. (1980). Channeling health: A review of televised health campaigns. *Health Education Quarterly, 7*(1), 56–89.

Maccoby, N., & Solomon, D. (1981). Heart disease prevention: community studies: In R. Rice & W. Paisley (Eds.), *Public communication campaigns* (pp. 105–125). Beverly Hills, CA: Sage.

Maloney, S. K. & Hersey, J. C. (1984). Getting messages on the air: Findings from the 1982 Alcohol Abuse Prevention campaign. *Health Education Quarterly, 11*(3), 273–292.

Manoff, R. K. (1985). *Social marketing: New imperative for public health*. New York: Praeger.

Milio, N. (1986). *Promoting health through public policy*. Ottawa: Canadian Public Health Association.

Minnesota Institute of Public Health (1988). *Market analysis profile 1986–1988*. Anoka, MN.

National Institutes of Health. (1982). *Pretesting in health communications: Methods, examples, and resources for improving health messages and materials*. Bethesda, MD: National Cancer Institute (NIH Pub. No. 83–1493).

National Institutes of Health (1983). Request for research grant applications: NIH-NCI-DRCCA-OD-83-10—Development and evaluation of smoking prevention and cessation interventions using the mass media. *NIH Guide for Grants and Contracts, 12*(8).

O'Keefe, G. J., & Reid-Nash, K. (1986). *The uses and effects of public service announcements*. Paper presented to the Midwest Association for Public Opinion Research annual conference, Chicago, IL.

Paisley, W. J. (1981). Public communication campaigns: The American experience: In R. E. Rice & W. J. Paisley (Eds.), *Public communication campaigns* (pp. 15–40). Beverly Hills, CA: Sage.

Perry, P. (1988). *Frontlines: Hopes are high, results low for the street workers at war with AIDS*. Unpublished manuscript, Gannett Center for Media Studies, New York.

Puska, P., Tuomilehto, J., Salonen, J., Neittaammaki, L., Maki, J., Virtumo, J., Nissinen, A., Koskela, K., & Takalo, T. (1979). Changes in coronary risk factors during a comprehensive five-year community program to control cardiovascular diseases (North Karelia Project). *British Medical Journal, 2*, 1173–1178.

Robertson, L. S., Kelly, A. B., O'Neill, B., Wixom, C. W., Eiswirth, R. S., & Haddon, W. (1974). A controlled study of the effect of television messages on safety belt use. *American Journal of Public Health, 64*(11), 1071–1080.

Rogers, E. M. (1973a). Mass media and interpersonal communication: In I. de Sola Pool, F. Frey, W. Schramm, N. Maccoby, & E. B. Parker (Eds.), *Handbook of communication* (pp. 290–310). Chicago: Rand McNally.

Rogers, E. M. (1973b). *Communication strategies for family planning*. New York: The Free Press.

Rogers, E. M., & Storey, J. D. (1987). Communication campaigns. In C. R. Berger & S. H. Chaffee (Eds.), *Handbook of communication science* (pp. 817–846). Beverly Hills, CA: Sage.

Rosenstock, I. M. (1974). Historical origins of the health belief model. *Health education monographs, 2*, 354–385.

Solomon, D. S. (1982). Health campaigns on television: In D. Pearl, L. Bouthilet, & J. Lazar (Eds.), *Television and behavior* (pp. 308–321). Rockville, MD: National Institite of Mental Health.

Stewart, A. (1986). The design of print for health education—principles for communication: In D. S. Leathar, G. B. Hastings, K. M. O'Reilly, & J. K. Davies (Eds.), *Health education and the media II* (pp. 23–29). Oxford: Pergamon Press.

Udry, J. R. (1974). *The media and family planning*. Chapel Hill: University of North Carolina Press.

U.S. will mail AIDS advisory to all households. (1988, May 5). *The New York Times*, p. B10.

Wallack, L. M. (1981). Mass media campaigns: The odds against finding behavior change. *Health Education Quarterly, 8*(3), 209–260.

Wallack, L. M. (1984). Social marketing as prevention: Uncovering some critical assumptions: In T. C. Kinnear (Ed.), *Advances in consumer research* (Vol. 11, pp. 682–687). Provo, UT: Association for Consumer Research.

Warner, K. E. (1977). The effects of the anti-smoking campaign on cigarette consumption. *American Journal of Public Health, 67,* 645–650.

Warner, K. E. (1979). Clearing the airwaves: The cigarette ad ban revisited. *Policy Analysis, 5,* 435–450.

Warner, K. E. (1981). Cigarette smoking in the 1970s: The impact of the anti-smoking campaigns on consumption. *Science, 211,* 729–731.

Warner, K. E. (1987). Television and health education: Stay tuned. *American Journal of Public Health, 77*(2), 140–142.

Worden, J. K., Flynn, B. S., Geller, B. M., Chen, M., Shelton, L. G., Secker-Walker, R. H., Solomon, D. S., Solomon, L. J., Couchey, S., & Costanza, M. C. (1988). Development of a smoking prevention mass media program using diagnostic and formative research. *Preventive Medicine, 17.*

World Health Organization. (1983). New approaches to health education in primary health care. *Technical reports series 690.* Geneva, Switzerland.

10

The Chronically Uninformed:
Closing the Knowledge
Gap in Health

Vicki S. Freimuth
University of Maryland

Health communicators often are confronted with the challenge of reaching target groups of low-income and poorly educated individuals because these low socioeconomic (SES) groups are frequently at higher risk for many health problems. Yet when these same campaigns are evaluated, these groups usually emerge as less exposed, less knowledgeable, and less likely to change their behaviors. In fact, there is some evidence that health communication campaigns actually increase the knowledge gaps between the "haves" and "have nots." This chapter identifies the critical issues that must be faced to communicate effectively with these "chronically uninformed." The first section of the chapter describes the health status of these low SES groups. In the second section, the knowledge gap hypothesis is reviewed as a possible explanation for the lack of information in these groups. The final section of the chapter suggests potential ways to reduce the knowledge gap.

DESCRIPTION OF THE HEALTH STATUS
OF LOW SES GROUPS

Bergner and Yerby (1968) presented a vivid description of the general health status of the poor.

> The poor behave differently from the middle class and the affluent across a wide spectrum related to health care. Illness is defined differently. There is less accurate health information. The poor are less inclined to

take preventive measures, and delay longer in seeking medical care. When they do approach health practitioners, they are more likely to select subprofessionals or the marginal practitioners often found in their neighborhoods. (p. 543)

According to a 1984 Census report, these economically disadvantaged persons include nearly 34 million Americans, 23 million Whites, 9.5 million Blacks, and 1.2 million of other races. Of these poor, over 3 million are persons 65 years and older and more than 1 million are migrant agricultural workers. The following is a list of different groups Childers and Post (1975) included in their description of the poor:

Mexican-Americans, Puerto Ricans, and other Spanish-speaking people;

American Indians and Eskimos;

Poor Black Americans and Whites;

Appalachians;

Poor farmers;

Migrant workers;

and Aging adults.

Although not all minority group members are poor, they are overrepresented in the lower SES groups. Although only 8.6% of all Whites were below the poverty level in 1983, 35.6% of all Blacks and 30% of all U.S. Hispanics fell into this low SES classification (National Cancer Institute, 1988). Moreover, minorities often suffer disproportionately from many serious health problems. Blacks, for example, have higher rates of heart disease, lung cancer, and diabetes than Whites. The infant mortality rate is still twice as high for Blacks as for Whites. Although comprising 12% and 6% of the U.S. population, respectively, Blacks and Hispanics account for 25% and 14% of all diagnosed cases of AIDS (Centers for Disease Control, 1986). Although only 15% of American children under 13 are Black, 54% of the children with AIDS are Black.

A special report from the American Cancer Society (ACS, 1985) showed that a person's chances of surviving one chronic disease, cancer, have more to do with economic status than with racial or ethnic background. In fact, the report revealed that the poor have a relative cancer survival rate of 10% to 15% lower than more affluent groups. In addition, the poor often have greater risk factors such as smoking, poor nutrition, and exposure to health hazards in the workplace. For example, smoking is a health risk that affects the disadvantaged more than the rest of society. Smoking is most common among the less educated and the less successful. Of men in professional and technical fields, 26% smoke, whereas 50% of men in blue-collar jobs smoke. Hall (1985) suggested that the disadvantaged do not have the same information or do not have the same ability to make choices. He reported that whereas 12% of teenagers planning to go to college smoke, 27% of teenagers not planning to attend college smoke.

The poor and minorities have less knowledge about many diseases. White adolescents in a San Francisco high school were more knowledgeable than Black adolescents about the cause, transmission, and prevention of AIDS, and Black adolescents were more knowledgeable than their Latino peers. Black and Latino adolescents were approximately twice as likely as White adolescents to have misconceptions about the casual transmission of AIDS (DiClemente, Boyer, & Morales, 1988). A positive correlation between education and knowledge of AIDS persisted even within a group of Black adolescent focus group participants from the District of Columbia (Center for Population Options, 1988). Students appeared to be much more informed than dropouts and older teens appeared more informed than younger ones.

Childers and Post (1975) summarized the four major problems related to the health information environment of disadvantaged adults:

1. They tend to know less about diseases—warning signals, symptoms, communicability.
2. They tend not to know about preventive health services, such as prenatal care, dental care, or health insurance.
3. They tend not to know where to turn for health services in general, and they do not know which specific services are available.
4. Folk-medicine—both the formal kind, like shamanism, and the informal kind, like backwoods herbal pharmacology—is well entrenched among the nonurban disadvantaged (pp. 44–45).

THE KNOWLEDGE GAP HYPOTHESIS

Health communicators have often turned to the mass media to reach these low-educated and poor groups with health information, but the results frequently have been disappointing. The knowledge gap hypothesis offers some explanation for these disappointing results. Historically, studies of mass media effects have demonstrated that education correlates strongly with acquisition of knowledge about public affairs and science from mass media. Tichenor, Donohue, and Olien (1970) formalized this observation in the knowledge gap hypothesis that predicts that as mass media information is infused into a social system, members with more education acquire knowledge faster than do those with relatively less education. Consequently, the gap in knowledge between the two social groups increases rather than decreases. Predictions are made for both one-time and multiple measurements:

1. Over time, acquisition of knowledge of a heavily publicized topic will proceed at a faster rate among better educated persons than among those with less education; and

2. At a given point in time, there should be a higher correlation between acquisition of knowledge and education for topics less highly publicized (Tichenor et al., 1970, p. 165).

The knowledge gap hypothesis includes three variables: level of mass media publicity in a particular setting, level of individuals' education, and level of individuals' knowledge about a specific subject. Time may be included as a fourth variable. Yet the term *knowledge gap* appearing in the literature may have several different meanings. In Gaziano's (1983) review of over 58 studies of the knowledge gap, she found it important to distinguish among the following meanings of the knowledge gap: (a) gaps found at one point in time, (b) gaps that may occur over time and may change in magnitude, (c) gaps that refer only to the relationship between education and knowledge without reference to media, and (d) gaps that result from media treatment or media exposure. Gaziano (1983) concluded from her review that most of the research supported the proposition that the higher the education, the greater the knowledge of various topics. This relationship does not directly support the original knowledge gap hypothesis, however, because the level of mass media publicity for topics is not considered. Gaziano's (1983) conclusion from time-trend studies actually reversed the original knowledge gap hypothesis. She concluded that increasing levels of media publicity may reduce gaps but that several other factors may be equally or more influential in narrowing gaps. Additional evidence refuting the knowledge gap comes from one-time case studies where the frequent finding of moderately sized gaps may indicate that media publicity played a part in decreasing initially larger gaps.

Gaziano (1983) analyzed several varying characteristics of the 58 studies to determine what other variables might have affected the knowledge gap. She found that the most frequent characteristics associated with knowledge inequalities seem to be type of topic and geographic scope of topic studied. Gaps are more likely to occur when (a) topics are international and national issues, (b) topics are of greater interest to high socioeconomic status (SES) persons than to low SES individuals, and (c) knowledge is conceptualized in civics class or textbook terms. Gaps occur less often or are smaller when topics are local and are likely to appeal to lower SES strata. There is only limited evidence to help us decide whether health topics fit this pattern.

First, there are several studies that support the existence of gaps in health knowledge at one point in time. Gaziano (1983) identified several knowledge gap studies of health topics and found that, although people of all educational backgrounds tend to be highly interested in health matters, they may still show knowledge disparities. Butler and Paisley (1976) also argued that health knowledge is unequally distributed throughout society, pointing out that health knowledge "haves" are young, White, and better educated, whereas the "have nots" are old, nonWhite, and less educated. Stojanovic's (1972) study of the awareness of Medicare supported this racial difference in knowledge. He found that the proportion of Black respondents who were unaware of the program was four times as great as Whites. In their study of the Minnesota Heart Health Program, Lee, Kline, Jacobs, and Hannan (1985) examined individual antecedents, family antecedents, and community antecedents to health knowledge and found that educational attainment and involvement in health were the most significant predictors of health knowledge.

There is less consistency with previous research on the way media publicity may affect gaps. Tichenor and his associates (1970) supported the original knowledge gap hypothesis with their 1968 research in two Minnesota cities, measuring recall of medical, biological, and social science topics in the news, and comparing recall to previous amount of newspaper publicity given to these subjects. On the other hand, Ettema, Brown, and Luepker (1983) failed to support the original knowledge gap hypothesis but did support Gaziano's conclusion that media publicity played a part in decreasing initially larger gaps. In their study of the effects of an informational campaign on cardiovascular health, Ettema and his associates (1983) found that the campaign virtually eliminated the existing gap between more and less well-educated segments. They identified motivation as a significant factor mediating gap effects. Based on limited research in the health area, it seems reasonable to conclude that, at any one time, there usually is a gap in the levels of knowledge about most health topics but that increasing the mass media information disseminated about that topic may reduce the gap.

Several alternative explanations have been suggested for the knowledge gap phenomenon. These explanations can be grouped under three categories: those that attribute the knowledge gap to characteristics of the audience, the message, and the social system.

Audience Characteristics

Tichenor and his colleagues' (1970) approach to causation is consistent with what other authors have called the individual blame bias (e.g., Rogers, 1983). They suggest that the "information haves" can be described as having:

1. Superior communication skills such as reading and comprehension.
2. Greater stored information, increasing awareness and capacity to understand new information.
3. More relevant social contacts who are likely to discuss the issues.
4. Selective exposure, acceptance, and retention to messages that follow from these previous differences.

Childers and Post (1975) suggest that the information universe of disadvantaged people is characterized by barriers that contribute to a knowledge gap. One of the first barriers for these people is the level of processing skills at their command. Reading ability is often quite low. English may be a second language. These disadvantaged people may have little experience in the communication skills we take for granted, such as bargaining for a car or negotiating a contract on a house.

Second, the disadvantaged are often locked into an information ghetto. Their information system is a closed one—any contact from the outside usually comes through the mass media, a one-way flow of information. As a result, much misinformation is prevalent. Internally generated information is accepted and disseminated similarly to other communities. But, as Childers and Post (1975) said, "there is a kind of social embargo against a great body of externally generated information" (p. 33).

The third major barrier among the disadvantaged is a fatalistic predisposition. Most research on the poor portrays them as despairing, fatalistic people with a pervasive sense of helplessness. Locus of control has been another popular construct used to describe this predisposition. Disadvantaged people are more likely to exhibit an external locus of control, meaning that their lives are controlled by outside forces over which they have little control. Niemi and Anderson (1971) described this predisposition differently. They speak of a "lower-class value stretch" in which these people do not abandon the general values of society but they generate an alternative set of values rationalized to fit their status. Certainly the disadvantaged are not as likely as the rest of society to change the undesirable conditions of their lives, or to see information as an instrument of their salvation.

The way the disadvantaged use available channels of communication is another barrier. As is the case with all of us, the disadvantaged have access to both informal and formal sources of information and prefer the informal sources to meet specific information needs. When the disadvantaged person does perceive a need for information and seeks it, there is evidence that the search is less intense (Childers & Post, 1975).

The other consistent conclusion in information channels studies, is the low level of readership among the disadvantaged. For example, Block (1972) studied mass media exposure patterns of Blacks in St. Louis and found that 40% did not read at all or less than 1 hour per week. Yet these same respondents rated newspapers as the most important information source, TV second, friends third, and advice from social workers as last. In a public opinion survey of a Black ghetto in Pittsburgh in 1967, 72% reported reading only a small portion of the newspaper but very few reported using it for news.

Television is always reported as the source most frequently used by the poor. It is unclear, however, whether television is being used for entertainment or for information. Olien, Donohue, and Tichenor (1978) found that as education went up, preferences for newspapers increased and preferences for television went down. Parker and Paisley's (1966) explanation for these findings was that education increases the need for information and reduces the need for escape.

Childers and Post (1975) reported a classification of information as either "ends" information or "means" information. The former relates to what you want to achieve and the latter relates to how to achieve it. The electronic media contain more "ends" information and the print media more "means" information. Childers and Post (1975) described the dilemma created by the overreliance of the disadvantaged adult on the electronic media: "He is overexposed to 'ends' information through television and radio, and sorely underexposed to the kind of information that might help him achieve the ends that he desires" (p. 40).

Childers and Post (1975) summarized their review of the information poor with this portrait of the disadvantaged adult in his natural information habitat:

Does not know which formal channels to tap in order to solve his problems, or what specific programs exist to respond to his needs.

Watches many hours of television daily, seldom reads newspapers and magazines and never reads books.

Does not see his problems as information needs.

Is not a very active information seeker, even when he does undertake a search.

May lean heavily on formal channels of information if it becomes apparent that the informal channels are inadequate and if his need is strongly felt.

Is locked into an informal information network that is deficient in the information that is ordinarily available to the rest of society. (pp. 42–43)

These audience factors need to be examined in light of what Ettema and Kline (1977) described as the difference versus the deficit thesis. The deficit thesis arose from research examining the achievement gap that assumed that the relationship between SES and intellectual performance was caused by a deficiency of basic cognitive ability. On the other hand, the difference thesis argues that people from different social strata have the same underlying competence as those in the mainstream of the dominant culture, "difference in performance being accounted for by the situations and contexts in which the competence is expressed" (Ettema & Kline, 1977, p. 186). An emphasis on deficits such as lack of communication skills to explain the knowledge gap predicts that gaps will always widen and never narrow. By contrast, the difference thesis predicts that

gaps widen in those circumstances in which lower SES persons are less motivated to acquire the information or in which the information is less functional for them, while gaps may narrow (and perhaps even fail to materialize in the first place) when the motivation to acquire the information is increased among the lower SES persons or when the information is functional for them. (Ettema & Kline, 1977, p. 188)

Ettema et al. (1983) believed that interest or motivation rather than education is the key mediating factor in the knowledge gap. Genova and Greenberg (1979) also found composite interest (a combination of social and self-interest) to be a better predictor of knowledge than education.

In a later study, Ettema (1984) further supported his argument for interest or motivation outweighing SES as an antecedent of information gain. He found that innovativeness and ability to see the importance of information was more important than SES. The ability to see the importance of information was positively related to system use while family income was negatively related. Moreover, use itself was most strongly related to reported benefits. Dervin (1980) also supported the difference perspective on audience factors when she challenged the construct validity of the knowledge gap because of its underlying traditional model of source-receiver. She favored instead the relativist model that underlies information seeking and uses and gratifications. Finally, there is the perspective promoted by McKnight (1985), which argues that the problem with lack of knowledge and utilization stems not from lack of information but from a mistrust and even a deliberate rejection of the "establishment" position.

In summary, audience causal factors can be grouped under those consistent with a deficit or a difference perspective. The difference perspective is more useful because it suggests opportunities to narrow or eliminate gaps. The necessary strategy appears to be making the information interesting and functional as well as credible for the specific audience.

Message Characteristics

Message characteristics affecting the knowledge gap have usually been discussed as some type of ceiling or upper limits in the knowledge to be disseminated. Ettema and Kline (1977) identified three types of ceilings that often appear in the literature on the knowledge gap: artifacts, imposed ceilings, and true ceilings. Artifacts refer to those ceilings that are only measurement artifacts that may be responsible for data showing lower SES individuals catching up. Cooke and his associates (1975) cited the "Sesame Street" evaluation as an example of the artifact type of ceiling. These authors claim that the measurements used were more sensitive to pre- to posttest improvements by children who scored lower initially than by children who scored higher on the pretest.

Two types of imposed ceilings were described by Ettema and Kline (1977): those imposed by the message itself and those imposed by the audience on itself. Those ceilings imposed by the message itself occur when the message is simple and limited, and, because the more informed audience members are likely to already have the information, the message allows the less informed audience members to catch up. There is evidence, for example, that the campaigns with the simple message that smoking is harmful to your health have reached nearly everyone and no significant knowledge gap remains. (This is certainly not to suggest that the behavior change has followed the knowledge gain.) The other category of imposed ceilings includes those imposed by the audience upon itself. Although this type of ceiling is not mentioned directly in the literature, Ettema and Kline (1977) reinterpreted results from a study of family planning and adolescents: Better informed adolescents felt that they had enough information and, thus, were not motivated to seek any more, giving less-informed adolescents a chance to catch up.

The final type of ceiling, the true ceiling, occurs when the knowledge being disseminated has a definite boundary. Once the "early knowers" have reached this boundary, there is an opportunity for the "later knowers" to catch up. Dramatic news events, such as the assassination of a public figure, are often given as examples of these true ceilings.

When there is a source-imposed ceiling or a true ceiling, gaps should narrow. Similarly, gaps will narrow when the higher SES audience members impose a ceiling on themselves and the lower SES members do not.

Message ceilings already are widely used in the health field to reduce knowledge gaps. Health communicators often develop campaign objectives with a type of ceiling imposed (i.e., they reduce the complexity of the desired behavior to its simplest form, e.g., "Don't smoke. Smoking is harmful to your health," and "Wear seat belts. They may save your life").

Social System Characteristics

Social system causal factors reflect the shift from individual blame to social system blame. Attributing gaps to the social system rather than the individual also reinforces the appropriateness of the difference thesis over the deficit thesis. Several authors (e.g., Olien, Tichenor, & Donohue, 1982; Tichenor, Donohue, & Olien, 1980) contend that structural variables must be considered (i.e., that the most important knowledge sources were more accessible to the most educated people). For example, these authors argued that it is the nature of the media that most science and public interest information is carried by print that is more available to high status people.

Ettema (1984) outlined places in the social system where gaps can develop:

1. *Development of the system*—Systems are often created and made available to specialized users who are already information rich (e.g., videotext users, personal health information systems.) The development of systems has been left to the private sector that determines who will have access and that generally is the higher SES groups. This problem is less significant in the health area because many information systems are developed by the public rather than the private sector.

2. *Adoption of the system*—Adopters tend to be relatively young, better

educated, and have an ability to see the information value of the system. Moreover, the desire to adopt the system may reflect less of a need for the information than a desire for it.

POTENTIAL WAYS TO REDUCE THE KNOWLEDGE GAP

Existing research on these low SES populations may not be adequate for planning health communication campaigns. There is much disparity in how different studies define low SES, by education, by income, by occupation, or some combination of these categories. Moreover, much of the research uses ethnicity, instead of one of these variables and there is no indication of social class differences. Better needs assessment studies must be built into the earliest phases of campaign planning so that messages can be targeted specifically and appropriately to the groups at highest risk. In addition to the traditional objectives of needs assessments to describe the target groups' demographics, health status, and knowledge, attitudes, and practices regarding the disease, this research also should determine the motivational appeals that might be effective with this audience. Several approaches to this motivational assessment are available in the literature (e.g., Carter et al., 1986; Simmons, 1988).

Each of these causal factors implies ways to reduce the knowledge gap. Audience communication skills could be improved as a way of overcoming deficits contributing to the knowledge gap. Literacy programs would be one example, as well as campaigns that attempt to teach fundamental processes as well as specific behavioral patterns. For example, campaigns for family planning could attempt to teach the basic reproductive cycle so that the information poor's foundation of knowledge could be improved.

The content of messages must be simple and concrete and, wherever possible, emphasize immediate rather than long-term benefits. The messages must be adapted sensitively to the target audience's cultural beliefs. A message developed for White general public audiences cannot simply be translated into Spanish and be effective with Hispanic audiences. Holly Smith, the information director of the San Francisco AIDS Foundation, reinforces the difficulty of reaching all groups in a community with a single campaign. She said, "For example, with Latinos, you try to reach family structures and health providers. With Blacks, you have to communicate through the churches, and with gays of course you need the bars" (Leishman, 1987, p. 55).

The audience's lack of interest in the topic or the low functional value of the information could be built into the campaign strategy so that part of the message is designed to stimulate interest and illustrate the functional value of the behaviors advocated.

The traditional emphasis on disseminating information through printed pamphlets and brochures, particularly when these print materials demand reading skills at a high school level or higher, is not likely to be effective with this group of infrequent readers. It has been argued that television is the potential knowledge leveler. Shingi and Mody (1976) found that TV could narrow the knowledge gap in a third world culture if the low knowledge people are given access and encouragement to watch, technical language is simplified, and highly credible sources are used, and if the information is presented as salient and appealing to the targeted audience. Other innovative channels also could be tried. Direct mail, for example, could be used to eliminate the lack of access some low SES people have to other media. Finnegan and Loken (1985) found that direct mail had a catch-up effect for males and lower educated groups. In addition, they found that using a personalized letter was more effective than a glossy brochure. In an unprecedented effort to reach all Americans with AIDS prevention information, the Centers for Disease Control (CDC) have implemented this strategy by mailing an informational brochure to every home in the United States. Telephones are another channel that can be used to reach people with health information. The Cancer Information Service, a regional network of offices reached by dialing 1-800-4 CANCER, where cancer questions are answered by knowledgeable staff, has been quite successful using this medium.

In addition to mass-mediated channels, informal channels in the community can be used to help reduce gaps. Kurtz (1968) identified nine roles potentially played by community members that are sources of interventions: worker, dweller, church member, manager, patient, welfare client, organization, legal, and mass media consumer. In a similar vein, Bergner and Yerby (1968) recommend the use of community health aides, untrained women who go out and ring doorbells as medical missionaries. These women should be intentionally untrained according to Bergner and Yerby (1968) because if trained they become too professional and become part of the institutional authority.

An unusual example of this type of community outreach has been used to reach intravenous drug users with AIDS prevention information. These addicts are a particularly difficult group to reach. Message strategies that use fear of the deadly effects of AIDS are unlikely to be effective because drug users already face the threat of death with every injection. Many addicts already tolerate poor health as a result of their addiction. Because intravenous drug users often are outside the mainstream of society, normal mass media or interpersonal channels will not reach them. Several programs have hired former addicts to visit "shooting galleries" in inner cities frequented by IV drug users to distribute bleach to sterilize used needles along with information about AIDS.

Credibility of sources is extremely important. The information must be disassociated with the White establishment bureaucracy that is so mistrusted by this social class. In the District of Columbia two community-based education groups have been formed with government money to reach out to the Black and Hispanic communities with AIDS information—Spectrum ("See the Light") for the majority Black population and Alianza ("An Effort from All for All") for the Hispanic group. Information from these two community groups should be more acceptable to the target audiences than information from the government.

The social system constraints cannot be ignored. If you expect people to adopt safer sex practices, you must be willing to communicate explicitly what those practices are and how to perform them. Moreover, if you expect IV drug users to abstain in order to protect themselves from AIDS, you need to increase the drug treatment facilities to accommodate the long lines waiting to be admitted. And, if you encourage certain high-risk groups to get tested for AIDS antibodies, you must provide low-cost, confidential, and convenient test facilities as well as long-term medical and social support for those who test positively.

SUMMARY

The focus of this chapter was on low SES groups who are notoriously less knowledgeable about most health issues. The dilemma for health communicators is that this group frequently is a priority target audience because it has higher incidence and mortality from many diseases.

Low SES groups often are less healthy. They are less inclined to take preventive measures, they delay longer in seeking medical care, and are likely to get medical care from clinics, emergency rooms, or marginal practitioners found in their neighborhoods. Consequently, their survival rates for many diseases are below those for more affluent Americans.

The knowledge gap hypothesis predicts that as mass media information is infused into a social system, members with more education acquire knowledge faster than do those with relatively less education. When the knowledge gap hypothesis is applied to health topics, only part of the hypothesis appears to be supported. Gaps in health knowledge do appear between low and high SES groups at one point in time.

However, increasing mass media information disseminated about that topic actually may reduce, instead of increase, the gaps.

The knowledge gap hypothesis has been attributed to characteristics of the audience, the message, and the social system. The audience of information "have nots" can be described as having inferior communication skills, an inadequate foundation of knowledge on which to expand, and fewer social network links. Message characteristics are usually discussed as some sort of ceiling or upper limit on the information that allows the information "have nots" to catch up. Social system causal factors shift the responsibility for the gaps from the individual to the social system. Design and accessibility of the system are factors accounting for its use or nonuse.

The final section of the chapter examined potential ways of reducing the knowledge gap in health. The problem of inadequate communication skills can be confronted directly through programs to upgrade these skills, such as literacy training or through design of simple, concrete messages transmitted through channels other than print. White, bureaucratic spokespersons are not likely to be credible to these audiences. Instead, community leaders and homophilous persons can be effective message sources.

The social system barriers to advocated behavior have to be removed if our messages are to be effective. Low cost, convenient, and competent services must be made available and personnel trained to be sensitive to these groups of clientele.

The AIDS epidemic has forced health communicators to confront the challenge of reaching these chronically uninformed audiences. The priority target groups for AIDS information are homosexual and bisexual males, intravenous drug users, prostitutes, and prisoners, many of whom are Black and Hispanic. With a fatal disease such as AIDS, a knowledge gap cannot be tolerated.

REFERENCES

American Cancer Society. (1985). *Cancer in the economically disadvantaged.* New York: Author.

Bergner, L., & Yerby, A. S. (1968). Low income and barriers to use of health services. *New England Journal of Medicine, 278*(10), 541–546.

Block, C. E. (1972). Prepurchase search behavior of low-income households. *Journal of Retailing, 48*(1), 3–15.

Butler, M., & Paisley, W. (1976). The potential of mass communication and interpersonal communication for cancer control. In J. W. Cullen, B. H. Fox, & R. N. Isom (Eds.), *Cancer: The behavioral dimensions* (pp. 205–229). New York: Raven Press.

Carter, W. B., Beach, L. R., Inui, T. S., Kirscht, J. P., & Prodzinski, J. C. (1986). Developing and testing a decision model for predicting influenza vaccination compliance. *HSR: Health Services Research, 20*(6), 897–932.

Center for Population Options. (1988). *D.C. teenagers and AIDS: Knowledge, attitudes, and behavior.* Unpublished manuscripts, Center for Population Options, Washington, DC.

Centers for Disease Control. (1986). Acquired immunodeficiency syndrome (AIDS) among blacks and Hispanic-United States. *Morbidity and Mortality Weekly Report, 35,* 655–666.

Childers, T., & Post, J. A. (1975). *The information poor in America.* Metuchen, NJ: Scarecrow Press.

Cooke, T. D., Appleton, H., Connor, R. F., Shaffer, A., Tamkin, G., & Weber, S. J. (1975). *"Sesame Street" revisited.* New York: Russell Sage Foundation.

Dervin, B. (1980). Communication gaps and inequities: Moving toward a reconceptualization. In B. Dervin & M. J. Voight (Eds.), *Progress in communication sciences* (Vol. 2, pp. 73–112). Norwood, NJ: Ablex.

DiClemente, R., Boyer, C. B., & Morales, E. S. (1988). Minorities and AIDS: Knowledge, attitudes, and misconceptions among black and latino adolescents *American Journal of Public Health, 78*(1), 55–57.

Ettema, J. S. (1984). Three phases in the creation of information inequities: An empirical assessment of a prototype videotext system. *Journal of Broadcasting, 28*(4), 389–395.

Ettema, J. S., Brown, J. W., & Luepker, R. V. (1983). Knowledge gap effects in a health information campaign. *Public Opinion Quarterly, 47,* 516–527.

Ettema, J. S., & Kline, F. G. (1977). Deficits, differences, and ceilings: Contingent conditions for understanding the knowledge gap. *Communication Research, 4*(2), 179–202.

Finnegan, J., & Loken, B. (1985, May). *The effects of direct mail on health awareness and knowledge in community heart health campaigns.* Paper presented to the International Communication Association Convention, Honolulu, HI.

Gaziano, C. (1983). The knowledge gap: An analytical review of media effects. *Communication Research, 10*(4), 447–486.

Genova, B. K. L., & Greenberg, B. S. (1979). Interests in news and the knowledge gap. *Public Opinion Quarterly, 43*(1), 79–91.

Hall, H. (1985). Cancer and blacks: The second-leading cause of death. *Urban League Review, 9*(2), 26–31.

Kurtz, N. R. (1968). Gatekeepers: Agents in acculturation. *Rural Sociology, 33*(1), 64–70.

Lee, J., Kline, F. G., Jacobs, D. R., Jr., & Hannan, P. J. (1985, May). *Acquisition of health messages for different individual and family types in different communities.* Paper presented at the annual meeting of the International Communication Association, Honolulu, HI.

Leishman, K. (1987, February). Heterosexuals and AIDS. *The Atlantic Monthly,* pp. 39–58.

McKnight, J. L. (1985, May). *Where can health communication be found?* Paper presented to the International Communication Association Convention, Honolulu, HI.

National Cancer Institute. (1988). *Background paper for Hispanic communications plan.* Unpublished paper, National Cancer Institute, Bethesda, MD.

Neimi, J. A., & Anderson, D. V. (1971). *Television: A Viable Channel for Educating Adults in Culturally Different Poverty Groups?—A literature Review* (Rep. No. AC010111). Syracuse, NY: Syracuse University. (ERIC Clearinghouse on Adult Education No. ED 048550).

Olien, C. N., Donohue, G. A., & Tichenor, P. J. (1978). Community structure and media use. *Journalism Quarterly, 55,* 445–455.

Olien, C. N., Tichenor, P. J., & Donohue, G. A. (1982, March). *Structure, communication, and social power: Evolution of the knowledge gap hypothesis.* Paper presented at Sommatie Conference, Veldhoven, the Netherlands.

Parker, E. B., & Paisley, W. J. (1966). *Patterns of adult information seeking.* Stanford, CA: Stanford University, Institute for Communication Research. (ERIC ED010-294).

Rogers, E. M. (1983). *Diffusion of innovations* (3rd. ed.). New York: The Free Press.

Shingi, P. M., & Mody, B. (1976). The communication effects gap: A field experiment on television and agricultural ignorance in India. *Communication Research, 3*(2), 171–190.

Simmons, R. E. (1988, April). *Lessons from behavioral models: Improving AIDS health communication campaigns.* Paper presented at the Eastern Communication Association's Annual Conference, Baltimore, MD.

Stojanovic, E. J. (1972). The dissemination of information about medicare to low-income rural residents. *Rural Sociology, 37,* 253–260.

Tichenor, P. J., Donohue, G. A., & Olien, G. N. (1970). Mass media flow and differential growth in knowledge. *Public Opinion Quarterly, 34*(2), 158–170.

Tichenor, P. J., Donohue, G. A., & Olien, G. N. (1980). Conflict and the knowledge gap. In P. J. Tichenor (Ed.), *Community conflict and the press* (pp. 175–203). Beverly Hills, CA: Sage.

11

Communication and Health Education

Gary L. Kreps
Northern Illinois University

Health education is an important communication process where relevant health information is disseminated to those individuals who can best utilize such data to reduce health risks and to increase the effectiveness of health care (Kreps, 1988; Tones, 1986). Health education is a complex, multifaceted communication process (Rubinson & Alles, 1984). It involves a wide range of different communicators such as health-care providers, biomedical and behavioral researchers, educators and students (at the primary, secondary, collegiate, graduate, professional school, and postgraduate levels), health-care consumers, government officials, as well as mass media representatives and their audiences. Health educators employ a wide range of health communication strategies and utilize many different communication channels to effectively disseminate and influence the use of relevant health information (Kreps, 1985c).

Health education messages are disseminated in both formal and informal communication contexts. Health education is presented formally through health-care provider/consumer interactions, classroom instruction, and mass media programs developed specifically to accomplish health information dissemination goals, whereas informal health education emerges spontaneously in everyday communication contacts with family, friends, co-workers, and popular mass media that indirectly provide or even allude to health information. Through the combination of formal and informal health education channels a vast number of individuals participate in the provision and consumption of health information. This chapter examines the systemic functions of interpersonal communication in formal and informal health information dissemination, and suggests strategies for promoting effective health education in society. (See the chapters by Donohew and Brown for more extensive coverage of the role of mass media in health education.)

HEALTH INFORMATION AND HEALTH EDUCATION

Human communication processes enable communicators to gather and interpret pertinent environmental information providing rationale, context, and direction for interpersonal coorientation and cooperation. (Kreps, 1986; Thayer, 1968). The communication of relevant information is a central element of health and health care (Kreps & Thornton, 1984). Health information directs individual and conjoint behaviors toward the accomplishment of health evaluation and maintenance (Kreps, 1988). Human communication is the process by which key information about health and illness, health information, is accessed. Health information is gathered through communication to ascertain levels of individual health, and to direct health-preserving behaviors. Communication processes also enable relevant health information to be shared among health-care consumers and providers, enabling these members of the health-care system to elicit cooperation in coordinating health-related activities (Cassata, 1980).

Health information is an important asset for both health-care consumers and providers (Freimuth & Stein, 1987). Health information is used to evaluate and direct health-care activities by helping consumers and providers make their most effective health-care choices (Dervin, Harlock, Atwood, & Garzona, 1980; Simoni, Vargas, & Casillas, 1982). Consumer uses of information in health care include self-monitoring of health condition by gathering information through conscious and autonomic internal feedback mechanisms, seeking evaluation of health condition from relevant others, gathering information from others about how to achieve and maintain optimal levels of health, as well as to evaluate the adequacy of different health-care activities and direct future behaviors. Health-care providers gather information from clients about clients' experiences with and interpretations of their health problems to inform diagnosis and treatment, as well as to share information with other health-care providers in coordinating the interdependent provision of health-care activities. Human communication is the primary tool used to seek, process, and utilize key health information (Kreps, 1988).

FORMAL HEALTH EDUCATION

Formal health education occurs when health-care and health-science specialists disseminate relevant health information to those who need such information (usually to health-care consumers, but also to health-care providers and students). Formal health education is provided to consumers during patient education efforts by many different health-care specialists and practitioners (such as doctors, nurses, pharmacists, dentists, and therapists) when these professionals share relevant health information with their clients (Greenfield, Kaplan, & Ware, 1985; Redman, 1984). Patient education messages are presented to consumers by health-care providers during office visits and classes, when providers write and/or distribute health information media (such as books, articles, and pamphlets concerning health issues), as well as when providers make public and mass-mediated presentations about health and health care. Public health campaigns are also designed to provide specific groups of consumers with relevant health information. (For more information about the design and functions of public health campaigns see chapter 7.)

Health-care providers, students, and educators also comprise important formal audiences for health information dissemination concerning a wide range of current health issues such as clinical research findings, epidemiological research trends, government regulatory policy developments, new health-care insurance guidelines, and health-care delivery strategies. Current and future health-care professionals are provided with relevant health information by many different health educators such as medical and nursing school professors, in-house training and workshop leaders, and conference speakers (Kreps, 1988; Young, 1987). Health-care providers depend on a variety of communication media such as books, journals, professional conferences, and seminars to help them learn about the latest techniques for diagnosing and treating health problems (Haynes et al., 1986; Kreps, Hubbard, & DeVita, 1988).

Unfortunately, a large body of evidence suggests that because health-care information and technologies are expanding at such a rapid rate and medical publications and meetings are dramatically proliferating to disseminate advances in medical knowledge, it is difficult, perhaps impossible, for health-care providers and consumers to keep abreast of the latest relevant treatment information (Covell, Uman, & Manning, 1985; Day, 1975; Harlem, 1977; Haynes et al., 1986; Kreps & Thornton, 1984; Shands, Goff, & Goff, 1982). In current health-care practice there is often a serious information and knowledge gap between the medical research community, specialized practice community, general practice community, and health-care consumers

(Baker, 1979; Brenner & Logan, 1980; Feldman, 1966; Kreps, Ruben, Baker, & Rosenthal, 1985, 1987; Lievrouw, Rogers, Lowe, & Nadel, 1986; McIntosh, 1974; Siegal, 1982).

To promote effective health care, efforts must be made to ensure that there is minimal information gap between the health-science research community, the health-care treatment community, and the consumers of health-care services (Kreps et al., 1987; Siegal, 1982). Several health education programs have been designed to help health-care providers keep abreast of pertinent prevention, diagnostic, and treatment information. For example, the National Cancer Institute (NCI) has developed an innovative computer-based health education program to provide physicians with state-of-the-art cancer treatment information, the Physician Data Query (PDQ) cancer information system (Kreps, Hubbard, & DeVita, 1988). Additionally, the curricula in schools that train and accredit health-care providers, continuing medical and nursing education programs, in-service training programs in hospitals and clinics, and health-care literature indexing and delivery systems such as MEDLINE serve as important channels for health education that health-care providers use to access relevant health information.

Health education efforts are also designed to narrow the information gap between health-care providers and the public by keeping the public informed about pertinent health-risk prevention and health-care treatment issues. Cassata (1978) suggested that communication specialists can perform an important role in health information dissemination by directing, facilitating, and translating communications between health-care providers and consumers. In fact, several public health education efforts developed and/or implemented by communication specialists have applied communication knowledge to the dissemination of health information via interpersonal and mediated communication channels. For example, Evans and Clarke (1986) reported the uses of interactive videodiscs to help provide cancer patients with relevant health information; Freimuth and Stein (1987) described the Cancer Information Service's use of a toll-free telephone hotline network to provide the public with cancer information; Hawkins, Day, Gustafson, Chewning, and Bosworth (1982) described the use of an interactive computer program to provide adolescents with sensitive health information about birth control and sexually transmitted diseases; and McDonald (1986) proposed a very ambitious comprehensive multimedia, interactive Personal Health Information System using "printed material, audiotex (telephone access information system), video, videotex, microcomputer-based software, and interactive video" (p. 4) to provide individuals with key health information for self-screening, self-assessment, triage (determining the seriousness of health problems), self-management, referrals, self-exploration, education, and personal health planning.

INFORMAL HEALTH EDUCATION

A great amount of information about health and health care is also disseminated to the public informally in everyday life by friends, family members, educational institutions, and popular mass media. Informal health education generally develops in two different ways:

1. *Directed* informal health education involves the use of health information messages offered to people in normal conversations by acquaintances who do not have specialized health-care training or professional knowledge, such as when friends recommend health problem remedies for each other;

2. *Undirected* informal health education includes messages that do not refer specifically to health or health care, but contain embedded health information that can influence those perceiving the messages, such as the way popular media like novels, television and radio entertainment shows, or general magazine and newspaper articles represent people and the health-care behaviors they engage in.

   Undirected informal health education is also communicated interpersonally in popular stories and legends that allude to health and illness. Many popular stories become cultural legacies in families, communities, and organizations leading to culturally based health beliefs and folk remedies. For example, communication of culturally based health care themes concerning the medicinal value of certain foods, like chicken soup being "Jewish penicillin," or "an apple a day keeps the doctor away," or "feed a fever, starve a cold" provide the basis for the indoctrination of cultural group members' health beliefs.

Informal health education performs an important role in helping to establish and maintain culturally approved health-care beliefs and practices and is often presented metacommunicatively as a form of cultural socialization (Kreps, 1988, 1986). Informal communication networks are extremely powerful sources of health information because these networks are easily accessible, well utilized, and personally involving for most people. Unfortunately, there are many instances where the content of health information provided by informal information sources contradicts current health-care knowledge being disseminated through formal information sources. Popular knowledge about health and health care that contradicts accepted scientific knowledge, such as the unfounded claims about nutritionally naive fad diets or oversimplistic folk remedies for complex health-care problems, while occasionally effective on the short-run, often lead individuals to engage in unhealthy long-term health-care practices that can cause them harm and undermine their faith in the formal health-care system.

INTERDEPENDENCE OF FORMAL AND INFORMAL HEALTH EDUCATION

Formal and informal health education communicates both content and relationship aspects of health information (Kreps, 1988; Watzlawick, Beavin, & Jackson, 1967). Content information in health education concerns descriptive data about the nature of health and health care, whereas relationship information in health education conveys the level of concern, sensitivity, and power health educators feel toward their audiences. Content and relationship information are interdependent components of health information that must support each other in health education efforts to be successful. For example, competent content information in health education communications surrounded by insensitive relationship information will seldom effectively reach and influence its audience because the audience for the health education efforts may be insulted and put off by the way the health information is being presented. On the other hand, sensitively communicated (good relationship information), health education messages describing fallacious health information (poor content information), although likely to be influential are unlikely to promote public health.

In actual practice, formal health education efforts are most effective at presenting content information and least effective at presenting relationship information. Formal health education, because it is generally offered by knowledgeable health specialists, usually contains timely and accurate health information, yet the social distance and, at times, dehumanizing interaction between health-care providers and consumers (as well as between health-care educators and students) can undermine health education efforts by alienating the recipients of health information.

Conversely, informal health education efforts are most effective at presenting relationship information and least effective at presenting content information. Informal health education, because it usually derives from individuals who are not trained health specialists or from those whose primary purpose is not to disseminate health information, often contains unsubstantiated and erroneous health information. Yet, people are usually receptive to informal health education because the information sources are generally comfortable and familiar communication contacts for them. Freimuth and Stein (1987) clearly described this problem, "The public faces a dilemma in using interpersonal sources for health information. Those persons who have the most authoritative information are the least accessible to them. Consequently, the less authoritative but more approachable interpersonal sources are more likely to be used" (p. 15). To promote effective interpersonal dissemination of health information, formal health education sources must increase their effectiveness in communicating relationship information, whereas informal health education sources must increase their abilities to provide accurate and timely content information about health and health care.

HEALTH EDUCATION
AND PUBLIC HEALTH-RISK PREVENTION

Health information is a crucial element in a preventive approach to public health care because relevant health information empowers individuals to take charge of their own health (Kreps & Thornton, 1984). Fueled by rising medical costs and other factors, increasing emphasis in recent years has been placed on prevention and the self-management of health care (Kreps, Ruben, Baker, & Rosenthal, 1987; Rosen, 1976). Health information is an essential ingredient in health-risk prevention in that information is needed to educate health-care providers and the public about potential health risks, state-of-the-art prevention and treatment techniques, as well as how to best implement appropriate strategies for minimizing health risks. Health education is designed to promote enlightened health care and self-management of health care by providing consumers and providers with relevant health information. To the extent that such educational efforts are successful they can lead to prevention of health risks (O'Donnell & Ainsworth, 1984; Smillie, 1946).

Kreps et al. (1985) clarified the interdependent relationships between health information, health education, health promotion, and the prevention of health risks by identifying health education as the mediating communication process that provides health information to those individuals who need such information for promoting health and preventing health risks. From this systemic perspective on health education health information is viewed as the system input and health education is the system process that functions by transforming the system inputs into the desired system outputs of health promotion and health-risk prevention. Human communication is the central system process that energizes health education.

Health promotion, prevention, and the self-management of health care presume that the public has sufficient levels of health information, and the attitudes and skills necessary for the effective use of this information in the management of its own health care. A recent national survey of the American public found that primary-care physicians are Americans' most preferred source of health information, with 84% of the 1,250 persons surveyed identifying a discussion with their personal physician as their most useful source of health information (Kreps et al., 1987). This finding underscores the importance of ensuring that general practice physicians are well informed and well trained to effectively communicate relevant health information to their clients. Maibach and Kreps (1986), in a survey of primary-care physicians, found that although these providers were genuinely concerned with health education, communication barriers such as lack of training and skills in health education and counseling strategies were inhibiting their information-dissemination efforts. In fact, evidence is bountiful that current physician communication practices often fail to supply their patients with satisfactory levels of health information (Hess, Liepman, & Ruane, 1983; Newell & Webber, 1983; Orleans, George, Houpt, & Brodie, 1985; Relman, 1982; Wechsler, Levine, Idelson, Rohman, & Taylor, 1983).

To accomplish large-scale health promotion and health-risk prevention goals, health education efforts have to be well planned and implemented. There are five major steps in directing health education efforts (see Fig. 11.1), (Kreps et al., 1985). This model shows that the first step in health education is the identification of clear health education goals. For example, what is the desired impact of the health education effort (increased knowledge, changed behavior, improved attitudes)? The second step is to identify the relevant health information that should be disseminated to accomplish health education goals. The third step involves audience identification and analysis (whom is the message targeted to and what are the key characteristics of this audience?). The fourth step is to identify the most appropriate and effective communication media for disseminating the health information to the desired audience (mass media, intermediaries, or interpersonal channels). The last step is to establish assessment criteria and to formatively evaluate the impact of the health education effort, feeding this information back to update the prior steps of the health education effort. From a systems perspective, these five health education steps become interdependent functional components that collectively accomplish system processes,

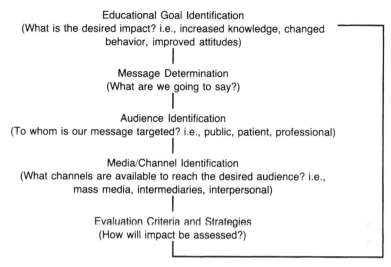

Educational Goal Identification
(What is the desired impact? i.e., increased knowledge, changed behavior, improved attitudes)

Message Determination
(What are we going to say?)

Audience Identification
(To whom is our message targeted? i.e., public, patient, professional)

Media/Channel Identification
(What channels are available to reach the desired audience? i.e., mass media, intermediaries, interpersonal)

Evaluation Criteria and Strategies
(How will impact be assessed?)

FIG. 11.1. Health education model.

transforming system inputs (health information) into desired system outputs (health promotion and health-risk prevention).

THE COMMUNICATION OF HEALTH EDUCATION

Health education is an extremely important part of health-care services. Health-care providers, like primary-care physicians, can improve the effectiveness of health-care delivery by informing consumers about health-care hazards, methods of self-evaluation, when and where to seek health-care services, and how to promote personal health. Health education can help empower health-care consumers to promote their own personal health and to direct their own care of the provision of relevant health information. Health education presentations can be used to provide relevant health information to both consumers and providers. Such presentations can be used as a means for improving health-care education by enhancing instructional communication and improving the quality of in-service training and education. Health-care practitioners can share information about new methods of patient care with their peers through their development of effective presentational speaking skills during in-service training sessions in their own health-care organizations (Kreps, 1981, 1982, 1985b; Young, 1987).

Optimally, health educators should be given training in presentational communication because they must develop the ability to present information on a wide range of different health-related topics to many different audiences with varying levels of knowledge about health and health care. Health education efforts are most effective when health-care providers develop the abilities to describe and explain complex health-care topics and procedures clearly and sensitively to patients, lay audiences, and professional groups (Kreps, 1985b, 1981; Kurtz, 1982). Health educators must be adept at audience analysis, possessing the ability to adapt messages to particular health education audiences by continually seeking and utilizing feedback. Informative and persuasive presentational speaking and writing skills are also important communication techniques for health educators to master. The abilities to effectively use persuasive strategies, data-gathering methods, topic organization, and delivery techniques are all crucial aspects of competent health education communication. The interplay of verbal and nonverbal messages in health information presentations must be skillfully coordinated for health education to be effective. Additionally, preparation and use of effective visual aids and graphics in presentations to clearly illustrate complex health topics will enhance health education efforts. Although health-care providers are the primary source of formal health education, health-care consumers should also be encouraged to develop effective presentational skills for informally educating family and friends about relevant health topics.

The effectiveness of interpersonally based patient education efforts is largely dependent on the abilities of health-care providers to competently communicate relevant health information to their clients; it depends on providers' development of effective communication skills (Kurtz, 1982; Redman, 1984). Unfortunately, current evidence suggests that many health-care providers are not adequately trained in communication skills to effectively disseminate health information to their clients (Hess et al., 1983; Kurtz, 1982; Lane, 1981; Maibach & Kreps, 1986; Relman, 1982). Communication and patient education training programs for health-care practitioners can help providers improve their abilities to supply their clients with relevant health information (Carroll & Monroe, 1980; Cline, 1983; Foley & Sharf, 1981; Kahn, Cohen & Jason, 1979; Kreps, 1988, 1985a, 1985b; Young, 1987).

RELATIONSHIP DEVELOPMENT AND HEALTH EDUCATION

Interpersonal communication plays an important role in health and health care. Effective interpersonal communication between people involved in health-care situations can help promote the delivery of high quality health information, whereas ineffective interpersonal health communication can seriously impair the quality of health-care education (Cline, 1983; Kreps & Thornton, 1984). It is at the interpersonal level of health communication that meaningful relationships are established between those individuals who are seeking and providing health-care services. Effective health-care relationships provide many health-related benefits, whereas the failure to establish satisfying relationships can cause many problems, hindering the accomplishment of health-care delivery goals (Cline, 1983; Kreps, 1988; Kreps & Thornton, 1984).

Relational partners use interpersonal communication to provide one another with information to evaluate individual health, exchange relevant information about health and health care, coordinate efforts, and share emotional support to help each other cope with health threats (Albrecht & Adelman, 1984, 1987; Kreps, 1988). Ineffective interpersonal health communication has been shown to lead to dissatisfaction with health-care services (Korsch & Negrete, 1972; Ruben & Bowman, 1986), alienation and breakdown in cooperation between health-care providers and consumers (Alpert, 1964; Blackwell, 1973; Caron, 1968; Hertz & Stamps, 1977; Lane, 1981), excessive interprofessional competition between interdependent health-care providers (Frank, 1961; Friedson, 1970), and can even have negative medical consequences on individuals that lead to premature death (Lynch, 1977).

The health-care interview is a relevant interpersonal communication setting for the exchange of messages between health-care providers and consumers, and the provision of relevant health information (Benjamin, 1981; Cline, 1983). An important communication function of the interview is to initiate the development of effective health-care relationships and the development of provider and consumer health communication roles. The messages that interview participants send one another establish the guidelines for an implicit contract between health-care provider and consumer (Kreps & Thornton, 1984). In effective interviews, care is taken by practitioners to put the patient at ease so they feel comfortable about sharing their perspective on personal health information and are receptive to health information provided to them, elicit full and clear information from the patient, maintain control of the interview by keeping it focused, maintain rapport with the patient by communicating in a sensitive and caring manner, and bring closure to the interview by responding to patient questions and clearly explaining future health-care activities the patient should engage in (Foley & Sharf, 1981). If the interview participants communicate effectively, the health-care interview can provide the interactants with a structured setting for establishing an effective provider/consumer relationship and gathering relevant health information (Carroll & Monroe, 1980; Kreps, 1985b). Medical school, nursing school, and other health professional educational programs must provide students with training in provider–patient communication and interviewing skills to facilitate effective information exchange in health-care interviews.

MISCOMMUNICATION AND HEALTH EDUCATION

Miscommunication, the misinterpretation of information communicated interpersonally, is an especially difficult health education problem (Kreps & Thornton, 1984). Miscommunication occurs in many different interpersonal communication situations because of the idiosyncratic ways individuals process information and create meanings. Miscommunications cause significant problems for health-care practitioners and clients because when they occur the intricate interdependent health-preserving behaviors these individuals engage in are guided by incorrect information. Miscommunications also lead consumers to misinterpret the health-care instructions explained to them by their providers, making it virtually impossible to comply with health-care instructions. Miscommunications also lead health-care providers to misinterpret messages their clients' provide them, resulting in incorrect diagnoses and inappropriate treatments. Mistakes stemming from provider/consumer miscommunications often have life or death consequences for health-care consumers (Kreps & Thornton, 1984).

There are several reasons why information misinterpretations happen quite frequently in health-care provider/patient interactions. Due to the complexity of health-care problems, diagnoses, and treatments, it is difficult to encode and decode health-care messages without ambiguities and information loss that lead to miscommunications. The overuse of medical jargon by health-care providers often confuses consumers of health care, leading to misinterpretations of practitioners' messages by patients (Barnlund, 1976; Woods, 1975). The urgency and emotionality of many health-care situations that often result in hastily encoded and decoded messages by both providers and consumers, also lead to miscommunications (Atman, 1972; Sethee, 1967). The differences in education and experience between practitioners and patients often lead to semantic distance between provider's and consumer's interpretations of interpersonal messages (Barnlund, 1976). Health-care consumers and providers must be trained to communicate clearly and seek feedback to avoid miscommunications (Kreps & Thornton, 1984). (For more information on the effects of miscommunications on health care see Chapter 3 by Thompson on interpersonal health communication.)

HEALTH COMMUNICATION EDUCATION

Many different communication problems and barriers that limit the effectiveness of health education efforts have been identified in the preceding sections of this chapter. Health communication training for health-care providers and consumers has been suggested as an important strategy for helping to resolve these problems and barriers. Effective health communication education will help health-care consumers and providers develop both knowledge and skills about communication in health care, helping consumers and providers develop health communication competencies (Cassata, 1978, 1980; Kreps, 1981, 1985a, 1985b; Kreps & Query, 1986; Kurtz, 1982; Ruben & Bowman, 1986).

To meet the health communication training needs of society educational institutions should implement curricula to help current and future health-care providers, as well as health-care consumers, develop both appreciation for the importance of effective communication in health education and enhanced abilities to communicate effectively in health-care situations (Barnlund, 1976; Cassata, 1980; Kreps, 1988). It is untenable to assume that health-care providers and consumers will develop adequate health communication skills and competencies on their own. Providers and consumers need support in developing knowledge and skills of competent health communication for use in seeking, interpreting, and providing relevant information to accomplish health education goals (Association of American Medical Colleges, 1984, 1985; Kreps & Query, 1986; Kurtz, 1982).

Health communication education can be implemented in several different ways. For example, in elementary and secondary schools, lessons for students about effective strategies for communicating about health problems (i.e., how to clearly describe a health problem they are experiencing, like pain, to others so they can get help) at home and in the health-care system, as well as informing students where they can get information about and help for their health problems can be integrated into basic health courses (Kreps, 1988). In pre-professional schools (like schools of medicine, nursing, pharmacy, dentistry, social work, etc.), health communication courses or course sections can complement and supplement existing courses for future health-care providers (Kahn et al., 1979; Kreps, 1982, 1985b; Kreps & Query, 1986; Kurtz, 1982). Continuing education programs for current health-care providers can offer seminars and workshops concerning health communication issues and the development of health communication competencies (Kreps, 1981; Ruben & Bowman, 1986; Young, 1987). College communication departments and schools can add communication courses to their undergraduate and graduate curricula to train communication students to become health communication specialists, as well as provide service courses for health-care profession students from their campuses and health care practitioners from their communities (Cassata, 1978; Kreps, 1981, 1982). College-based health communication courses can be most effective if they are designed to serve interprofessional groups of students, representing different parts of the health-care system (i.e., different health-care provider professions, consumers, and health-care system administrators) to promote the development of interprofessional understanding and cooperation in the delivery of health care (Hill, 1978; Kreps, 1985b, 1988; Kreps & Thornton, 1984).

Implementation of health communication curricula at each of these educational levels can help maximize health-care consumers' and providers' development of health communication competencies (Kreps, 1988; Kreps & Query, 1986). By increasing the communication competencies of health-care consumers and providers we can increase the effectiveness of formal and informal channels of health education in disseminating relevant health information to all segments of society. Better formal and informal dissemination of relevant health information can ultimately lead to increasing levels of public health by empowering individuals to choose the best available strategies for health promotion, helping to reduce levels of public morbidity and mortality.

REFERENCES

Albrecht, T., & Adelman, M. (1984). Social support and life stress: New directions for communication research. *Human Communication Research, 11,* 3–32.

Albrecht, T., & Adelman, M. (1987). *Communicating social support.* Newbury Park, CA: Sage.

Alpert, J. (1964). Broken appointments. *Pediatrics, 34,* 127–132.

Association of American Medical Colleges. (1984). *Physicians for the twenty-first century.* Washington, DC: Author.

Association of American Medical Colleges. (1985). Report of the working group on fundamental skills. *Journal of Medical Education, 59,* 125–134.

Atman, N. (1972). Understanding your patient's emotional response. *Journal of Practical Nursing, 22,* 22–25.

Baker, S. (1979). The diffusion of a high technology medical innovation: The computed tomography scanner example. *Social Science and Medicine, 13,* 155–162.

Barnlund, D. (1976). The mystification of meaning: Doctor-patient encounters. *Journal of Medical Education, 51,* 716–725.

Benjamin, A. (1981). *The helping interview* (3rd ed.). Boston: Houghton Mifflin.

Blackwell, B. (1973). Patient compliance. *New England Journal of Medicine, 289,* 249–252.

Brenner, D., & Logan, R. (1980). Some considerations in the diffusion of medical technologies: Medical information systems. In D. Nimmo (Ed.), *Communication yearbook 4* (pp. 609–623). New Brunswick, NJ: Transaction.

Caron, H. (1968). Patients' compliance with a medical regimen. *Journal of the American Medical Association, 203,* 922–926.

Carroll, J., & Monroe, J. (1980). Teaching clinical interviewing in the health professions: A review of empirical research. *Evaluation and the Health Professions, 3,* 21–45.

Cassata, D. (1978). Health communication theory and research: An overview of the communication specialist interface. In B. Ruben (Ed.), *Communication yearbook 2* (pp. 495–504). New Brunswick, NJ: Transaction.

Cassata, D. (1980). Health communication theory and research: A definitional overview. In D. Nimmo (Ed.), *Communication yearbook 4* (pp. 583–589). New Brunswick, NJ: Transaction.

Cline, R. (1983). Interpersonal communication skills for enhancing physician-patient relationships. *Maryland State Medical Journal, 32,* 272–278.

Covell, D. G., Uman, G. C., & Manning, P. R. (1985). Information needs in office practice: Are they being met? *Annals of Internal Medicine, 103,* 596–599.

Day, S. (1975). *Communication of Scientific Information.* New York: Karger.

Dervin, B., Harlock, S., Atwood, R., & Garzona, C. (1980). The human side of information: An exploration in a health communication context. In D. Nimmo (Ed.), *Communication yearbook 4* (pp. 591–608). New Brunswick, NJ: Transaction.

Evans, S. H., & Clarke, P. (1986, February). *Using the interactive videodisc to help cancer patients.* Paper presented to the Communicating With Patients Conference, Tampa, FL.

Feldman, J. (1966). *The dissemination of health information.* Chicago: Aldine.

Foley, R., & Sharf, B. (1981). The five interviewing techniques most frequently overlooked by primary care physicians. *Behavioral Medicine, 11,* 26–31.

Frank, L. (1961). Interprofessional communication. *American Journal of Public Health, 51,* 1798–1804.

Freidson, E. (1970). *Professional dominance: The social structure of medical care.* Chicago: Aldine.

Freimuth, V. S., & Stein, J. (1987, November). *The public's search for health information.* Paper presented to the Speech Communication Association Convention, Boston, MA.

Greenfield, S., Kaplan, S., & Ware, J. E. (1985). Expanding patient involvement in care: Effects on patient outcomes. *Annals of Internal Medicine, 102,* 520–528.

Harlem, D. (1977). *Communication in Medicine.* Paris: S. Karger.

Hawkins, R., Day, T., Gustafson, D., Chewning, B., & Bosworth, K. (1982, May). *Using computer programs to provide health information to adolescents.* Paper presented to the International Communication Association Convention, Boston, MA.

Haynes, R. B., McKibon, K. A., Fitzgerald, D., Guyatt, G. H., Walker, C. J., & Sackett, D. L. (1986). How to keep up with the medical literature: 1. Why try to keep up and how to get started. *Annals of Internal Medicine, 105,* 149–153.

Hertz, P., & Stamps, P. (1977). Appointment-keeping behavior re-evaluated. *American Journal of Public Health, 67,* 1033–1036.

Hess, J. W., Liepman, M. R., & Ruane, T. J. (1983). *Family practice and preventive medicine: Health promotion in primary care.* New York: Human Sciences Press.

Hill, S. K. (1978). Health communication: Focus on interprofessional communication. *Communication Administration Bulletin, 25,* 31–36.

Kahn, G. S., Cohen, B., & Jason, H. (1979). The teaching of interpersonal skills in U.S. medical schools. *Journal of Medical Education, 54,* 29–35.

Korsch, B., & Negrete, V. (1972). Doctor-patient communication. *Scientific American, 227,* 66–74.

Kreps, G. L. (1981, November). *Communication training for health care professionals.* Paper presented to the Speech Communication Association Convention, Anaheim, CA.

Kreps, G. L. (1982, May). *Health communication education: Retrospect and prospect for curricular development.* Paper presented to the International Communication Association Convention, Boston, MA.

Kreps, G. (1985a, April). *Interpersonal communication in health care: Promises and problems.* Paper presented to the Eastern Communication Association Conference, Providence, RI.

Kreps, G. (1985b, April). *The development and presentation of an interprofessional survey course in health communication.* Paper presented to the Eastern Communication Association Conference, Providence, RI.

Kreps, G. L. (1985c, October). *Health information, health education, and health promotion: Health communication with the public.* Paper presented to the Medical Communication Conference, James Madison University, Harrisonburg, VA.

Kreps, G. (1986). *Organizational communication: Theory and practice.* White Plains, NY: Longman.

Kreps, G. (1988). The pervasive role of information in health and health care: Implications for health communication policy. In J. Anderson (Ed.), *Communication yearbook 11* (pp. 238–276). Menlo Park, CA: Sage.

Kreps, G. L., Hubbard, S. M., & DeVita, V. T. (1988). The role of the Physician Data Query on-line cancer information system in health information dissemination. *Information and Behavior, 2,* 362–374.

Kreps, G. L., & Query, J. L. (1986, November). *Assessment and testing in the health professions.* Paper presented to the Speech Communication Association Convention, Chicago, IL.

Kreps, G. L., Ruben, B. D., Baker, M., & Rosenthal, S. (1987). A national survey of public knowledge about digestive health and disease: Implications for health education. *Public Health Reports, 102,* 270–277.

Kreps, G. L., Ruben, B. D., Baker, M., & Rosenthal, S. (1985, May). *Health information, education, and prevention: A national survey of public knowledge about digestive health and disease.* Paper presented to the International Communication Association Conference, Honolulu, HI.

Kreps, G. L., & Thornton, B. C. (1984). *Health communication: Theory and practice.* New York: Longman.

Kurtz, S. M. (1982, May). *A format for teaching information giving skills to health care professionals.* Paper presented to the International Communication Association Convention, Boston, MA.

Lane, S. (1981, November). *Interpersonal situation: Empathic communication between medical personnel and patients.* Paper presented to the Speech Communication Association Conference, Anaheim, CA.

Lievrouw, L. A., Rogers, E. M., Lowe, C. U., & Nadel, E. (1986, May). *Communication networks among biomedical scientists: Triangulation as a research methodology.* Paper presented at the International Communication Association Conference, Chicago, IL.

Lynch, J. (1977). *The broken heart: The medical consequences of loneliness.* New York: Basic Books.

Maibach, E. W., & Kreps, G. L. (1986, September). *Communicating with patients: Primary care physicians' perspectives on cancer prevention, screening, and education.* Paper presented to the International Conference on Doctor–Patient Communication, The Centre for Studies in Family Medicine, University of Western Ontario, London, Ontario, Canada.

McDonald, M. D. (1986, June). *The emergence of the personal health information system.* Paper presented to the Communication Technologies in Health Promotion Conference, National Cancer Institute, Bethesda, MD.

McIntosh, J. (1974). Process of communication, information seeking control associated with cancer: A selected review of the literature. *Social Science and Medicine, 8,* 167–187.

Newell, G. R., & Webber, C. F. (1983). The primary care physician in cancer prevention. *Family and Community Health, 5,* 77–84.

O'Donnell, M. P., & Ainsworth, T. H., (Eds.). (1984). *Health promotion in the workplace.* New York: Wiley.

Orleans, C. T., George, L. K., Houpt, J. L., & Brodie, K. H. (1985). Health promotion in primary care: A survey of U.S. family practitioners. *Preventive Medicine, 14,* 636–647.

Redman, B. K. (1984). *The process of patient education* (5th ed.). New York: Mosby.

Relman, A. A. (1982). Encouraging the practice of preventive medicine and health promotion. *Public Health Reports, 97,* 216–219.

Rosen, G. (1976). *Preventive medicine in the United States 1900–1975.* New York: Prodist.

Ruben, B. D., & Bowman, J. C. (1986). Patient satisfaction (Part 1): Critical issues in the theory and design of patient relations training. *Journal of Healthcare Education and Training, 1,* 1–5.

Rubinson, L., & Alles, W. F. (1984). *Health education: Foundations for the future.* St. Louis: Mosby.

Sethee, U. (1967). Verbal responses of nurses to patients in emotion-laden situations in public health nursing. *Nursing Research, 16,* 365–368.

Shands, V. P., Goff, L. D., & Goff, D. H. (1982, May). *Rx for OTC users: Improved health education.* Paper presented to the International Communication Association Convention, Boston, MA.

Siegel, E. R. (1982). Transfer of information to health practitioners. In B. Dervin & M. Voight (Eds.), *Progress in communication sciences* (Vol. 3, pp. 311–334). Norwood, NJ: Ablex.

Simoni, J. J., Vargas, L. A., & Casillas, L. (1982, May). *Medicine showmen and the communication of health information.* Paper presented to the International Communication Association Convention, Boston, MA.

Smillie, W. G. (1946). *Preventive medicine and public health.* New York: MacMillan.

Thayer, L. (1968). *Communication and communication systems: In organizations, management, and interpersonal relations.* Homewood, IL: Irwin.

Tones, B. K. (1986). Health education and the ideology of health promotion: A review of alternative approaches. *Health Education Research, 1,* 3–12.

Watzlawick, P., Beavin, J., & Jackson, D. (1967). *Pragmatics of human communication.* New York: W. W. Norton.

Wechsler, H., Levine, S., Idelson, R. K., Rohman, M., & Taylor, J. O. (1983). The physician's role in health promotion—A survey of primary care practitioners. *New England Journal of Medicine, 308*(2), 97–100.

Woods, D. (1975). Talking to people is a doctor game that doctors don't play. *Canadian Medical Association Journal, 113,* 1105–1106.

Young, L. (1987, November). *Inservice education in the nursing home setting.* Paper presented to the Speech Communication Association Convention, Boston, MA.

Author Index

Numbers in *italics* denote complete reference citation

A

Aaker, D.A., 87, *88*
Aasterud, M., 31, *45*
Abelman, R., 125, *133*
Abelson, R., 141, *152*
Adams, J.S., 103, 104, *105*
Adelman, M.B., 42, *45,* 75, *88,* 101, 102, 103, *105,* 197, *200*
Adler, K., 30, *45*
Aguilera, D.C., 40, *45*
Ainsworth, T.H., 193, *203*
Ajzen, I., 157, *168*
Albrecht, T.L., 42, *45,* 75, *88,* 102, *105,* 197, *200*
Albritton, W.L., 129, *133*
Aldrich, R.A., 44, *48*
Allaire, B., 57, 64, 65, *65*
Allen, J., 20, *22*
Allen, R.F., 20, *22*
Alles, W.F., 187, *203*
Allport, G.W., 52, *65*
Alpert, J., 197, *200*
Anderson, B.J., 40, *46*
Anderson, D.V., 176, *185*
Anderson, J.G., 102, *105*
Andrus, L.H., 71, *88*
Annyas, A.A., 30, *48*
Antonovsky, A., 75, *88*

Applton, H., 179, *185*
Argyle, M., 95, *105*
Arntson, P., 31, 34, *45,* 78, *88*
Aronoff, C., 125, *131*
Aronson, E., 100, *107*
Arthur, R.L., 75, *91*
Ashby, M., 34, 35, *46*
Atkin, C.K., 123, 124, 125, *131, 133,* 153, 161, 162, *167*
Atkin, R., 79, *90*
Atman, N., 198, *200*
Atwood, R., 37, *46,* 188, *201*
Austin, M.J., 77, *89*
Axelrod, M.D., 85, 87, *88*
Aydelotte, M.K., 41, *45*

B

Backer, T.E., 153, *167*
Backlund, P., 60, *68*
Baker, M., 60, *67,* 190, 193, 194, *202*
Baker, S., 189, *200*
Ball, R.A., 36, *49*
Bandura, A., 111, 128, *131,* 157, *167*
Baran, S.J., 125, *131*
Bargh, J.A., 137, 138, 140, 141, *149*
Barnard, D., 34, *45*
Barnes, G.P., 149, *149*

Subject Index

215

Printed and bound by CPI Group (UK) Ltd, Croydon, CR0 4YY

17/10/2024

01775687-0017